Renal Physiology

Bruce M. Koeppen, M.D., Ph.D.

Associate Professor of Medicine & Physiology
Associate Dean, Preclinical & Graduate Education
Division of Nephrology
University of Connecticut Health Center
Farmington, Connecticut

Bruce A. Stanton, Ph.D.

Associate Professor of Physiology
Department of Physiology
Dartmouth Medical School
Hanover, New Hampshire

Illustrations by
Peter P. Mitchell

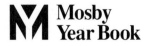

Mosby Year Book

St. Louis Baltimore Boston Chicago London Philadelphia Sydney Toronto

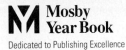
Mosby
Year Book
Dedicated to Publishing Excellence

Editor: Kimberly Kist
Assistant Editor: Penny Rudolph
Editorial Project Manager: Jolynn Gower
Production Assistant: Pete Hausler
Designer: David Zielinski

Printed in the United States of America

Mosby—Year Book, Inc.
11830 Westline Industrial Drive
St. Louis, Missouri 63146

Library of Congress Cataloging-in-Publication Data

Koeppen, Bruce M.
    Renal physiology / by Bruce M. Koeppen and Bruce A. Stanton :
illustrations by Peter P. Mitchell.
      p.   cm.
    Includes bibliographical references and index.
    ISBN 0-8016-6329-6
    1. Kidneys—Physiology. 2. Water-electrolyte balance (Physiology)
I. Stanton, Bruce A. II. Title.
    [DNLM: 1. Kidney—physiology. WJ 301 K78r]
QP249.K64 1992
612.4'63—dc20
DNLM/DLC
for Library of Congress   91-33720
                                            CIP

92 93 94 95 96 GW/GW/DC 9 8 7 6 5 4 3 2 1

Preface

To the instructor: This book is intended to provide students in the biomedical and health sciences with a basic understanding of kidney function. For the student at this stage, we feel it is better to master a few central concepts and ideas, rather than to assimilate a large array of facts. Consequently, this book is designed to teach the important aspects and fundamental concepts of normal renal function. Emphasis has been placed on presenting the material in a clear and concise manner. To accomplish this goal we have been selective in the material included. The broader field of nephrology, with its current and future frontiers, is better learned at a later time, and only after the "big picture" has been well established. For clarity and simplicity we have made statements as assertions of fact, even though we recognize not all aspects of a particular problem have been resolved.

To the student: As an aid to learning this material each chapter includes a list of objectives that reflect the fundamental concepts to be mastered. At the end of each chapter we have provided a list of key words and concepts that should serve as a check list while working through the chapter. We also have provided a series of self-study questions. These questions review the central principles to be mastered.

Because these questions are learning tools, answers and explanations are provided in an appendix. Finally, a comprehensive multiple choice exam is included at the end of the book. We recommend working through this test only after completing the book. In this way it can serve as an indicator of where additional work or review is required.

We have provided an annotated bibliography of selected books, monographs, and papers. This bibliography is highly selective and is intended to provide the next step in the study of the kidney; a place where details are added to the subjects presented here, and other aspects of the kidney not treated in this book are explored.

We encourage all who use this book to send us your comments and suggestions. Please let us know what we have done right, as well as what needs improvement.

Acknowledgments: We thank the following individuals who have read early versions of the book, and provided excellent criticism and suggestions: Drs. K. Conrad, P. Friedman, G. Giebisch, M. Knepper, J. Laycock, K. Madsen, E. Sigman, and P. Steinmetz. We also thank K. Majeski for her help in preparing the manuscript.

Bruce M. Koeppen
Bruce A. Stanton

Contents

INTRODUCTION TO THE KIDNEY, xv

1   Physiology of Body Fluids, 1

Objectives, 1
Physicochemical Properties of Electrolyte Solutions, 1
    Molarity and equivalence, 1
    Osmosis and osmotic pressure, 2
    Osmolarity and osmolality, 3
    Tonicity, 3
    Oncotic pressure, 5
    Specific gravity, 6
Volumes of Body Fluid Compartments, 6
Measurement of Body Fluid Volumes, 6
Composition of Body Fluid Compartments, 7
Fluid Exchange Between Body Fluid Compartments, 9
    Capillary fluid exchange, 9
    Cellular fluid exchange, 10
Key Words and Concepts, 13
Self-Study Study Problems, 13

2   Structure and Function of the Kidneys and the Lower Urinary Tract, 15

Objectives, 15
Structure of the Kidneys, 15
    Gross anatomy, 15
    Ultrastructure of the nephron, 16
    Ultrastructure of the glomerulus, 19
    Ultrastructure of the juxtaglomerular apparatus, 2\
    Innervation of the kidney, 24
Anatomy and Physiology of the Lower Urinary Tract, 24
    Gross anatomy and histology, 24
    Innervation of the bladder, 25
    Passage of urine from the pelvis to the bladder, 25
    Micturition, 25
Key Words and Concepts, 26
Self-Study Problems, 26

3   Glomerular Filtration and Renal Blood Flow, 27

Objectives, 27
Renal Clearance, 27
    Measurement of glomerular filtration rate—clearance of inulin, 29
    Filtration plus tubular reabsorption—clearance of glucose, 31
    Filtration plus tubular secretion—clearance of PAH, 32
    Measurement of renal plasma flow and renal blood flow, 33
    Using clearance to estimate transport mechanism, 37
Glomerular Filtration and Renal Blood Flow, 37
    Determinants of ultrafiltrate composition, 38
    Dynamics of ultrafiltration, 40
    Renal blood flow, 43
    Regulation of renal blood flow, 45
        Sympathetic control, 45
        Angiotensin II, 46
        Prostaglandins, 47
Key Words and Concepts, 47
Self-Study Problems, 47

4   Renal Transport Mechanisms: NaCl and Water Reabsorption Along the Nephron, 49

Objectives, 49
General Principles of Membrane Transport, 50
General Principles of Transepithelial Solute and Water Transport, 52
NaCl and Water Reabsorption Along the Nephron, 52
    Proximal tubule, 52
        NaCl and water reabsorption, 54
        Organic anion and organic cation secretion, 57
        Protein reabsorption, 58
    Henle's loop, 59
    Distal tubule and collecting duct, 62
Regulation of NaCl and Water Reabsorption, 65
    Starling forces, 65
    Glomerulotubular balance, 66
    Hormones, 68
    Sympathetic nervous system, 68
Key Words and Concepts, 68
Self-Study Problems, 68

5   Regulation of Body Fluid Osmolality, 70

Objectives, 70
Antidiuretic Hormone, 71
    Osmotic control of ADH secretion, 72
    Hemodynamic control of ADH secretion, 74
    ADH actions on the kidneys, 75
    Disorders of ADH secretion and action, 76
Thirst, 76
Countercurrent Multiplication by Henle's loop, 77
    Transport and permeability properties of the nephron segments, 79
    Medullary interstitial osmotic gradient, 79

Vasa recta function: countercurrent exchange, 82
Diuresis vs. antidiuresis and the role of ADH, 83
Integrated View of the Urine Concentrating Process, 83
Quantitating Renal Diluting and Concentrating Ability, 85
Key Words and Concepts, 88
Self-Study Problems, 89

6   Regulation of Extracellular Fluid Volume, 91

Objectives, 91
Concept of Effective Circulating Volume, 92
ECV Volume Sensors, 93
Vascular low-pressure volume receptors, 93
Vascular high-pressure volume receptors, 93
Volume Receptor Signals, 93
Renal sympathetic nerves, 93
Renin-angiotensin-aldosterone system, 94
Atrial natriuretic peptide, 97
Antidiuretic hormone, 97
Control of Na^+ Excretion with Normal ECV, 97
Mechanisms for keeping Na^+ delivery to the collecting duct constant, 99
Regulation of collecting duct Na^+ reabsorption, 100
Control of Na^+ Excretion with Increased ECV, 100
Control of Na^+ Excretion with Decreased ECV, 103
Edema and the Role of the Kidneys, 105
Alterations in Starling forces, 106
Capillary hydrostatic pressure (P_c), 106
Plasma oncotic pressure (Π_c), 106
Lymphatic obstruction, 106
Capillary permeability, 106
The role of the kidneys, 107
Key Words and Concepts, 108
Self-Study Problems, 108

7   Regulation of Potassium Balance, 110

Objectives, 110
Overview of K^+ Homeostasis, 110
Internal K^+ Distribution, 112
Epinephrine, 114
Insulin, 114
Aldosterone, 114
Acid-base balance, 114
Plasma osmolality, 114
Cell lysis, 115
Exercise, 115
External K^+ Balance: Excretion of K^+ by the Kidneys, 115
Cellular Mechanisms of K^+ Transport by the Distal Tubule and Collecting Duct, 117
Regulation of K^+ Excretion, 118
Plasma [K^+], 118
Aldosterone, 119

Flow rate of tubular fluid, 119
Antidiuretic hormone, 121
Acid-base balance, 121
$[Na^+]$ of tubular fluid, 122
Key Words and Concepts, 122
Self-Study Problems, 122

8   Regulation of Acid-Base Balance, 123
Objectives, 123
The CO_2/HCO_3^- Buffer System, 123
Metabolic Production of Acid and Alkali, 124
Overview of Renal Acid Excretion, 125
HCO_3^- Reabsorption Along the Nephron, 127
Regulation of HCO_3^- Reabsorption, 128
Formation of New HCO_3^-: The Role of Ammonia, 130
Response to Acid-Base Disorders, 132
Extracellular and intracellular buffering, 133
Respiratory defense, 134
Renal defense, 134
Simple Acid-Base Disorders, 135
Metabolic acidosis, 135
Metabolic alkalosis, 136
Respiratory acidosis, 136
Respiratory alkalosis, 136
Analysis of Acid-Base Disorders, 137
Key Words and Concepts, 138
Self-Study Problems, 138

9   Regulation of Calcium, Magnesium, and Phosphate Balance, 140
Objectives, 140
Ca^{++}, 140
Overview of Ca^{++} homeostasis, 141
Ca^{++} transport along the nephron, 142
Cellular mechanisms of Ca^{++} reabsorption, 143
Regulation of Ca^{++} excretion, 144
Mg^{++}, 144
Overview of Mg^{++} homeostasis, 145
Mg^{++} transport along the nephron, 146
Regulation of Mg^{++} excretion, 146
PO_4^{3-}, 147
Overview of PO_4^{3-} homeostasis, 147
PO_4^{3-} transport along the nephron, 149
Regulation of PO_4^{3-} excretion, 150
Key Words and Concepts, 151
Self-Study Problems, 151

10 Physiology of Diuretic Action, 152

Objectives, 152
General Principles of Diuretic Action, 152
 Sites of action of diuretics, 153
 Response of more distal nephron segments, 153
 Adequate delivery of diuretics to their site of action, 154
 Volume of the ECF, 154
Mechanisms of Action of Diuretics, 155
 Osmotic diuretics, 155
 Carbonic anhydrase inhibitors, 156
 Loop diuretics, 156
 Thiazide diuretics, 157
 K^+-sparing diuretics, 157
Effect of Diuretics on the Excretion of Water and Other Solutes, 158
 Solute-free water, 158
 K^+ handling, 159
 HCO_3^- handling, 160
 Ca^{++}, Mg^{++}, and PO_4^{3-} handling, 160
Key Words and Concepts, 162
Self-Study Problems, 162

ADDITIONAL READING, 164

Appendix A: ANSWERS TO SELF-STUDY PROBLEMS, 168

Appendix B: REVIEW EXAMINATION, 182

To Gerhard Giebisch, M.D., scientist, scholar, and teacher, who has been our mentor and good friend.

Introduction to the Kidney

The kidney presents in the highest degree the phenomenon of sensibility, the power of reacting to various stimuli in a direction which is appropriate for the survival of the organism; a power of adaptation which almost gives one the idea that its component parts must be endowed with intelligence.

E. Starling—1909

As recognized by Starling, the kidneys are viewed more appropriately as regulatory organs, rather than as excretory organs. However, it is clear that the excretory function of the kidneys is central to their ability to regulate the composition and volume of the body fluids.

In this book, various aspects of renal physiology are explored. Emphasis is placed on providing insight and understanding into the major functions of the kidneys. They are:

- regulation of body fluid osmolality and volume.
- regulation of electrolyte balance.
- regulation of acid-base balance.
- excretion of metabolic products and foreign substances.
- production and secretion of hormones.

In the chapters that follow these aspects of renal function are considered in detail. However, to provide a broad perspective and overview they are described briefly here.

Regulation of body fluid osmolality and volume (Chapters 1, 5 and 6): The kidneys are critical components of the system involved in the control of both the osmolality and volume of the body fluids. The control of body fluid osmolality is important for the maintenance of normal cell volume in virtually all tissues of the body, while control of the volume of the body fluids is necessary for normal function of the cardiovascular system. The kidneys, working in an integrated fashion with components of the cardiovascular and central nervous systems, accomplish these tasks by regulating the excretion of water and NaCl.

Regulation of electrolyte balance (Chapters 4, 5, 6, 7, 8, and 9): The kidneys play an essential role in regulating the amount of several important inorganic ions in the body including: Na^+, K^+, Cl^-, HCO_3^-, H^+, Ca^{++}, Mg^{++}, and PO_4^{3-}. The kidneys also contribute to the maintenance of organic ion balance. For example, the excretion of many of the intermediates of the Krebs cycle (e.g., citrate, succinate) is controlled by the kidneys. To maintain appropriate balance, the excretion of any one of these electrolytes must be balanced to the daily intake. If intake exceeds excretion, the amount of a particular electrolyte in the body increases. Conversely, if excretion exceeds intake, the amount decreases. For many of these electrolytes the kidneys are the sole or primary route for excretion from the body. Thus, electrolyte balance is achieved by carefully matching daily excretion by the kidneys with daily intake.

Regulation of acid-base balance (Chapter 8): Many of the metabolic functions of the body are exquisitely sensitive to pH. Thus, the pH of the body fluids must be maintained within very narrow limits. This is accomplished by buffers within the body fluids, and by the coordinated action of the lungs and kidneys. The importance of the kidneys in acid-base balance is underscored by the fact that acid accumulates in the body fluids of individuals with reduced renal function.

Excretion of metabolic products and foreign substances (Chapters 3 and 4): The kidneys excrete a number of end products of metabolism that are no longer needed by the body. These so-called waste products include urea (from amino acids), uric acid (from nucleic acids), creatinine (from muscle creatine), end products of hemoglobin metabolism, and metabolites of hormones. These substances are eliminated from the body by the kidneys at a rate that matches their production. Thus, their concentrations within the body fluids are maintained constant. The kidneys also represent an important route for elimination of foreign substances from the body including drugs, pesticides, and other chemicals ingested in the food. When renal function is compromised, metabolic waste products and foreign substances accumulate in the body because their excretion in the urine decreases. The accumulation of some of these substances is thought to be responsible for the symptoms associated with chronic renal failure.

Production and secretion of hormones (Chapters 6 and 9): The kidneys are important endocrine organs producing and secreting renin, 1,25-dihydroxyvitamin D_3, and erythropoietin. Renin activates the renin-angiotensin-aldosterone system, which is important in regulating blood pressure, as well as sodium and potassium balance. 1,25-dihydroxyvitamin D_3 is necessary for normal reabsorption of Ca^{++} by the gastrointestinal tract, and for its deposition in bone. With renal disease, the ability of the kidneys to produce 1,25-dihydroxyvitamin D_3 is impaired, and levels of this hormone are reduced. As a result, Ca^{++} reabsorption by the intestine is decreased. This reduced intestinal Ca^{++} reabsorption contributes to the abnormalities in bone formation seen in patients with chronic renal disease. Erythropoietin stimulates red blood cell formation by the bone marrow. With many kidney diseases erythropoietin production and secretion is reduced. Decreasing erythrocyte production is a causal factor in the anemia seen in chronic renal failure.

In the following chapters various aspects of these important renal functions are considered. Where information is available, these functions are considered at several levels of organization: whole kidney, single nephron, individual tubular cell, cell membrane, and transport protein.

1 Physiology of Body Fluids

▪ OBJECTIVES

1. Identify the major body fluid compartments, their volumes, and their ionic compositions.
2. Explain the principle involved in using a marker to measure the volume of a fluid compartment and how this is used to measure the volumes of the various body fluid compartments.
3. Describe the following properties of solutions:
   a. Osmotic pressure
   b. Osmolarity and osmolality
   c. Oncotic pressure
   d. Tonicity
4. Recognize the forces responsible for movement of water across cell membranes and the capillary endothelium.
5. Calculate changes in the volumes of the intracellular and extracellular fluid compartments that result from shifts in fluid between these compartments under various pathophysiological conditions.

O ne of the major functions of the kidney is to maintain the volume and composition of the body fluids despite wide variation in the daily intake of water and solutes. In this chapter, the volume and composition of body fluids is discussed to provide a background for the study of the kidney as a regulatory organ. Some of the basic principles, terminology, and concepts related to the properties of solutes in solution are also reviewed.

▪ PHYSICOCHEMICAL PROPERTIES OF ELECTROLYTE SOLUTIONS

Molarity and Equivalence

The amount of a substance dissolved in a solution (i.e., its concentration) is expressed either in terms of *molarity* or *equivalence*. Molarity is the amount of a substance relative to its molecular weight. For example, glucose has a molecular weight of 180 g/mole. If 1 L of water contains 1 g of glucose, the molarity of this solution would be determined as:

$$\frac{1 \text{ g/L}}{180 \text{ g/mole}} = 0.0056 \text{ moles/L or } 5.6 \text{ mmol/L} \tag{1-1}$$

For uncharged molecules, such as glucose and urea, concentrations in the body fluids are usually expressed in terms of molarity. Because many of the substances of biological interest are present at very low concentrations, units are more frequently expressed in the millimolar range (mmol/L or mM).

The concentration of solutes, which normally dissociate into more than one particle when dissolved in a solution (e.g., NaCl), is usually expressed in terms of equivalence. Equivalence refers to the stoichiometry of the interaction between cation and anion, and is determined by the valence of these ions. For example, con-

1

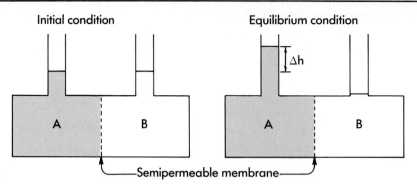

Figure 1-1 ■ Schematic representation of osmotic water movement, and the generation of an osmotic pressure. The solute particles in compartment A cause water to move by osmosis from compartment B across the semipermeable membrane into compartment A. The water column in compartment A will rise (Δh) until the hydrostatic pressure generated by the water column stops the flow of water from compartment B into compartment A. This hydrostatic pressure is equal to the osmotic pressure generated by the solute particles in compartment A.

sider a 1-L solution containing 9 g of NaCl (molecular weight = 58.4 g/mole). The molarity of this solution, according to equation 1-1, is 154 mmol/L. Because NaCl dissociates into Na^+ and Cl^- ions, and assuming complete dissociation, this solution contains 154 mmol/L of Na^+ and 154 mmol/L of Cl^-. Since the valence of these ions is 1, these concentrations can also be expressed as milliequivalents (mEq) of the ion per liter (i.e., 154 mEq/L for Na^+ and Cl^- respectively).

For univalent ions such as Na^+ and Cl^-, concentrations expressed in terms of molarity and equivalence are identical. However, this is not true for ions having valences greater than 1. Accordingly, the concentration of Ca^{++} in a 1-L solution containing 0.1 g of this ion would be expressed as:

$$\frac{0.1 \text{ g/L}}{40.1 \text{ g/mole}} = 2.5 \text{ mmol/L} \qquad (1\text{-}2)$$

$$= 2.5 \text{ mmol/L} \times 2 \text{ Eq/mole} = 5 \text{ mEq/L}$$

Although some exceptions exist, it is customary to express concentrations of ions in milliequivalents per liter.

Osmosis and Osmotic Pressure

The movement of water across cell membranes occurs by the process of *osmosis*. The driving force for this movement is the osmotic pressure difference across the membrane. Figure 1-1 illustrates the concept of osmosis and the measurement of the osmotic pressure of a solution.

Compartment A and compartment B are separated by a semipermeable membrane (i.e., the membrane is highly permeable to water, but impermeable to solute). Compartment A contains a solute, and compartment B contains only distilled water. Over time, water will move by osmosis from compartment B to compartment A.* This will raise the level of fluid in compartment A (Δh) and decrease the level in compartment B. At equilibrium, the hydrostatic

---

*This water movement is driven by the concentration gradient for water. Because of the presence of solute particles in compartment A, its concentration of water is less than that in compartment B. Consequently, water moves across the semipermeable membrane from compartment B to compartment A down its gradient.

pressure exerted by the column of water will stop the movement of water from compartment B to compartment A. This pressure will be equal and opposite to the osmotic pressure exerted by the solute particles in compartment A.

Osmotic pressure is a colligative property of a solution, which is determined solely by the number of solute particles in that solution. It is not dependent upon such factors as the size of the solute particles, their mass, or chemical nature (e.g., valence). Osmotic pressure, measured in atmospheres (atm), (Π) is calculated by *van't Hoff's law* as:

$$\Pi = nCRT \qquad (1\text{-}3)$$

where

n = Number of dissociable particles per molecule

C = Total solute concentration

R = Gas constant

T = Temperature in degrees Kelvin ($^\circ$K)

For a molecule that does not dissociate in water, such as glucose or urea, a solution containing 1 mmol/L of the solute at 37° C can exert an osmotic pressure of:

$$\Pi = (1)(0.001 \text{ mol/L})(0.082 \text{ atm L/mol }^\circ\text{K}) \qquad (1\text{-}4)$$
$$(310 \, ^\circ\text{K}) = 2.54 \times 10^{-2} \text{ atm}$$

Because 1 atmosphere equals 760 mm Hg at sea level:

$$\Pi = (760 \text{ mm Hg/atm})(2.54 \times 10^{-2} \text{ atm}) = \qquad (1\text{-}5)$$
$$19.3 \text{ mm Hg}$$

Alternatively, osmotic pressure is expressed in terms of osmolarity (see below). Thus, a solution containing 1 mmol/L of solute particles exerts an osmotic pressure of 1 milliosmole/L (1 mOsm/L).

For substances that dissociate in a solution, n of equation 1-3 will have a value other than 1. For example, a 150 mmol/L solution of NaCl has an osmolarity of 300 mOsm/L because each molecule of NaCl dissociates into an Na^+ and a Cl^- ion (i.e., n = 2). If dissociation of a substance into its component ions is not complete, n will not be an integer. Accordingly, osmolarity for any solution can be calculated as:

$$\text{Osmolarity} = \text{Concentration} \times \qquad (1\text{-}6)$$
$$\text{Number of dissociable particles}$$
$$\text{mOsm/L} = \text{mmole/L} \times \text{Particles/mole}$$

Osmolarity and Osmolality

Osmolarity and osmolality are frequently confused and incorrectly interchanged. *Osmolarity* refers to the number of solute particles per 1 L of water, while *osmolality* is the number of solute particles in 1 kg of water. For dilute solutions, the difference between osmolarity and osmolality is insignificant. However, measurements of osmolarity are temperature-dependent, because the volume of water varies with temperature (i.e., the volume is larger at higher temperatures). In contrast, osmolality, which is based on the mass of water, is temperature-independent. For this reason, osmolality is the preferred term for biological systems and is used throughout this and subsequent chapters. Osmolality has the units of Osm/kg H_2O. Because of the dilute nature of physiological solutions, osmolalities are expressed in the range of milliosmoles per kilogram of water (mOsm/ kg H_2O).

Table 1-1 shows the relationships between molecular weight, equivalence, and osmoles for a number of physiologically significant solutes.

Tonicity

The *tonicity* of a solution is related to its effect on the volume of a cell. Solutions that do not change the volume of a cell are said to be *isotonic*. A *hypotonic* solution causes a cell to swell, while a *hypertonic* solution causes a cell to shrink. Although related to osmolality, tonicity also takes into consideration the permeability of a solute across a cell membrane.

Consider two solutions: a 150 mmol/L solution of NaCl and a 300 mmol/L solution of urea.

Table 1-1 ■ Units of measurement for physiologically significant substances

Substance	Atomic/molecular weight	Equivalents/mole	Osmoles/mole
Na^+	23.0	1	1
K^+	39.1	1	1
Cl^-	35.5	1	1
HCO_3^-	61.0	1	1
Ca^{++}	40.1	2	1
PO_4^{3-}	95.0	3	1
NH_4^+	18.0	1	1
NaCl	58.5	2[a]	2[b]
$CaCl_2$	111	4[c]	3
Glucose	180	—	1
Urea	60	—	1

a. One equivalent each for Na^+ and Cl^-.
b. NaCl does not dissociate completely in solution. However, throughout the text we assume complete dissociation does occur.
c. Ca^{++} contributes two equivalents, as do the Cl^- ions.

Both solutions have an osmolality of 300 mOsm/kg H_2O (the number of dissociable particles per molecule is 2 for NaCl and 1 for urea), and therefore are isosmotic. When red blood cells are placed in the two solutions, those in NaCl maintain their normal volume, while those placed in urea swell and eventually burst. Thus, the NaCl solution is isotonic and the urea solution is hypotonic. The differential effect of these solutions on red blood cell volume is related to the permeability of the plasma membrane to NaCl and urea.

To exert an osmotic pressure across a membrane, a solute must not permeate that membrane. Because urea is highly permeable across the red blood cell membrane, it cannot exert an *effective osmotic pressure* to balance that generated by the intracellular solutes of the red blood cell.* Consequently, driven by the os-

motic pressure of the intracellular solutes, water is drawn into the cell, and the cell swells. In contrast, NaCl remains outside of the cell and exerts an effective osmotic pressure opposite to that generated by the contents of the red blood cell. As described in a subsequent section, Na^+ and Cl^- can cross the cell membrane and enter the cell, but they are expelled from it by specific membrane transporters.

To take into account the effect of a solute's membrane permeability on osmotic pressure, it is necessary to rewrite equation 1-3 as:

$$\Pi = \sigma(nCRT) \qquad (1\text{-}7)$$

where sigma (σ) is a measure of the relative permeability of a solute across a cell membrane.

For a solute that is freely permeable across a cell membrane, such as urea, $\sigma = 0$, and no osmotic pressure is exerted. Such a substance is said to be an *ineffective osmole*. In contrast, $\sigma = 1$ for a solute that is impermeable across a cell membrane. These solutes are termed *effective osmoles*. Many solutes are neither freely permeable nor completely impermeable across cells membranes ($0 < \sigma < 1$) and will generate an osmotic pressure that is only a fraction of

*Urea traverses the plasma membrane of red blood cells via a specific transport protein, with the driving force for movement being the urea concentration gradient. The transport protein simply facilitates the movement of urea from one side of the membrane to the other. Urea is only freely permeable across membranes containing this urea transporter.

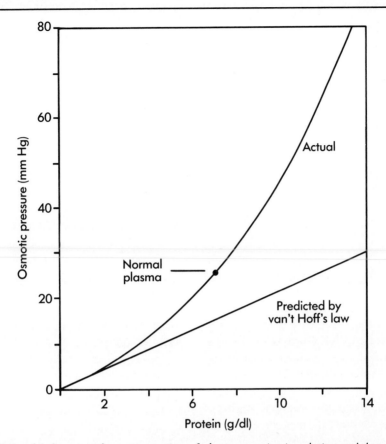

Figure 1-2 ■ Relationship between the concentration of plasma proteins in solution and the osmotic pressure (oncotic pressure) they generate. Protein concentration is expressed as g/dl. Normal plasma protein concentration is indicated. Note how the actual pressure generated exceeds that predicted by van't Hoff's Law.

what is expected from the total solute concentration.

Oncotic Pressure

Oncotic pressure is the osmotic pressure generated by large molecules (especially proteins) in a solution. As illustrated in Figure 1-2, the magnitude of the osmotic pressure generated by a solution of protein does not conform to van't Hoff's law. The cause of this anomalous relationship between protein concentration and osmotic pressure is not completely understood, but appears to be related to the size and shape of the molecule. For example, the correlation

to van't Hoff's law is more precise with small, globular proteins than with larger protein molecules.

The oncotic pressure exerted by proteins in plasma has a normal value of approximately 25 mm Hg. Although this pressure is small when compared with osmotic pressure (a solution having an osmolality of 1 mOsm/kg H_2O exerts an osmotic pressure of 19.3 mm Hg), it is a force for fluid movement across capillary membranes, especially the glomerulus (see Chapter 3). Oncotic pressure is not a major force when considering the movement of water across cell membranes.

Specific Gravity

The total solute concentration in a solution can also be measured as *specific gravity*. Specific gravity is the weight of a volume of solution divided by the weight of an equal volume of distilled water. Thus, the specific gravity of distilled water is 1 g/ml. Because biological fluids contain a number of different substances, their specific gravities are greater than 1 g/ml. For example, normal plasma has a specific gravity in the range of 1.008-1.010 g/ml.

The specific gravity of urine is commonly measured in the clinical setting and used to assess the concentrating ability of the kidney. The specific gravity of urine varies in proportion to its osmolality. However, because specific gravity depends on the number of solute particles and their weight, the relationship between specific gravity and osmolality is not always predictable. For example, patients who have been injected with radiocontrast dye (molecular weight > 500) for x-ray studies can have high values of urine specific gravity (1.040-1.050 g/ml), even though the urine osmolality is similar to that of plasma (300 mOsm/kg H_2O).

■ VOLUMES OF BODY FLUID COMPARTMENTS

Water makes up approximately 60% of the body's weight, with variability among individuals being a function of the amount of adipose tissue. Because the water content of adipose tissue is lower than that of other tissues, increased amounts of adipose tissue reduce the fraction of total body weight due to water. The percentage of body weight attributed to water also varies with age. In newborn infants, it is approximately 75%. This decreases to the adult value of 60% by the age of 1 year.

As illustrated in Figure 1-3, *total body water* is distributed between two major compartments, which are divided by the cell membrane.* The *intracellular fluid (ICF)* compartment is larger and contains approximately two thirds of the total body water. The remaining one third is contained in the *extracellular fluid (ECF)* compartment. Expressed as percentages of body weight, the volumes of total body water, ICF, and ECF can be estimated as:

Total body water = 0.6 × (Body weight)

ICF   = 0.4 × (Body weight)

ECF   = 0.2 × (Body weight)

The extracellular fluid compartment is subdivided into *interstitial fluid* and *plasma,* which are divided by the capillary endothelium. The interstitial fluid surrounds the cells in the various tissues of the body and composes three fourths of the extracellular fluid volume. Included in this compartment is water contained within the bone and dense connective tissue. Plasma represents the remaining one fourth of the extracellular fluid volume.

■ MEASUREMENT OF BODY FLUID VOLUMES

The volume of a body fluid compartment can be measured by adding a "marker" to the compartment and measuring its concentration once equilibrium has been reached. For example, if 5 g of a marker is added to a beaker of water of unknown volume and, after equilibration, the concentration of this marker in the beaker is 10 g/L, the volume of water in the beaker is:

$$\text{Volume} = \frac{\text{Amount}}{\text{Concentration}} = \frac{5 \text{ g}}{10 \text{ g/L}} = 0.5 \text{ L} \qquad \textbf{(1-8)}$$

To be an effective marker of a particular body fluid compartment, a substance must be confined to and evenly distributed throughout that com-

---

*In these and all subsequent calculations, it is assumed that 1 L of fluid (e.g., ICF and ECF) has a mass of 1 kg. This allows interconversion between units of osmolality and volume.

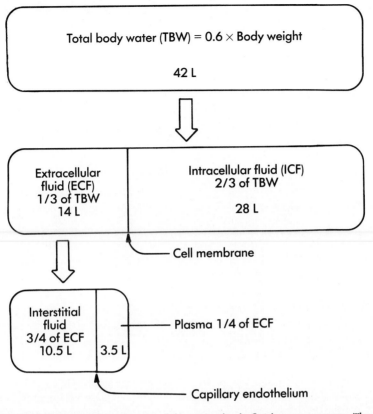

Figure 1-3 ■ Relationship between the volumes of the major body fluid compartments. The actual values shown are calculated for a 70 kg individual.

Table 1-2 ■ **Substances used as markers for body fluid compartments**

Body fluid compartment	Marker
Total body water	Tritiated water
Extracellular fluid	Inulin, mannitol
Plasma	^{3}H-albumin, Evans blue

No marker exists for the intracellular fluid compartment; its volume is calculated as the difference between total body water and extracellular fluid volumes.

partment. In addition, the marker should be physiologically inert, not metabolized, and easily measured. Table 1-2 lists some markers that have been used to measure the volumes of the various body fluid compartments. Note that no marker measures the intracellular fluid volume; this volume is calculated as the difference between total body water and the extracellular fluid.

In practice, measuring the volumes of body fluid compartments is complicated, because markers are excreted from the body while they are distributed throughout the compartments. However, it is possible to make appropriate corrections by quantifying the amount excreted (see self-study problems).

■ **COMPOSITION OF BODY FLUID COMPARTMENTS**

The concentrations of the major cations and anions in the ECF are illustrated in Figure 1-4. Na^+ is the major cation of the ECF, and Cl^- and

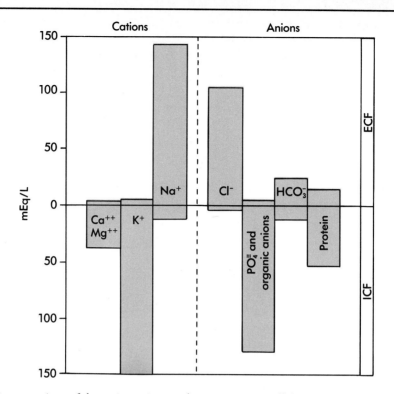

Figure 1-4 ■ Concentrations of the major cations and anions in extracellular (ECF) and intracellular (ICF) fluids. The concentrations of Ca^{++} and Mg^{++} are the sum of these two ions. Concentrations represent the total of free and complexed ions. The total concentration of cations equals that of anions in both compartments.

HCO$_3^-$ are the major anions. The ionic composition of the interstitial fluid and plasma in the ECF is similar, because these compartments are separated only by the capillary endothelium, a barrier that is freely permeable to small ions. The major difference between interstitial fluid and plasma is that the latter contains significantly more protein. This differential concentration of protein can affect the distribution of cations and anions between the two compartments, as plasma proteins have a net negative charge and tend to increase the cation concentrations and reduce the anion concentrations in the plasma compartment. However, this effect is small, and the ionic compositions of the interstitial fluid and plasma can be considered to be identical.

Because of its abundance, Na$^+$ (and its attendant anions, primarily Cl$^-$ and HCO$_3^-$) is the major determinant of ECF osmolality. Accordingly, a rough estimate of ECF osmolality can be obtained by simply doubling the sodium concentration [Na$^+$]. For example, if the plasma [Na$^+$] is 145 mEq/L, the osmolality of plasma and ECF can be estimated as:

Plasma osmolality = 2(Plasma [Na$^+$]) =   (1-9)
    290 mOsm/kg H$_2$O

Because water is in osmotic equilibrium across the capillary endothelium and the plasma membrane of cells, measurement of plasma osmolality also provides a measure of ECF and ICF osmolality.

The composition of ICF is more difficult to

measure and can vary significantly from one tissue to another. Figure 1-4 provides information on the intracellular composition. In contrast to ECF, the $[Na^+]$ of ICF is extremely low. K^+ is the predominant cation of this compartment. The asymmetric distribution of Na^+ and K^+ across the plasma membrane is maintained by the activity of the ubiquitous $Na^+ - K^+ - ATPase$. By its action, Na^+ is expelled from the cell in exchange for K^+.

The anion composition of ICF also differs markedly from that of ECF, with the $[Cl^-]$ of ICF lower in comparison. The major ICF anions are phosphates, organic anions, and protein.

■ FLUID EXCHANGE BETWEEN BODY FLUID COMPARTMENTS

Water moves freely between the body fluid compartments. Two forces determine this movement: hydrostatic pressure and osmotic pressure. While hydrostatic pressure from the pumping of the heart and osmotic pressure by plasma proteins (oncotic pressure) are important determinants of fluid movement across the capillary endothelium, only osmotic pressure differences between ICF and ECF cause fluid movement across cell membranes.

Capillary Fluid Exchange

The movement of fluid across the capillary endothelium is determined by the algebraic sum of the hydrostatic and oncotic pressures as expressed by the following equation *(Starling forces):*

$$\text{Fluid movement} = K_f[(P_c + \Pi_i) - (P_i + \Pi_c)] \quad (1\text{-}10)$$

where

K_f = Filtration coefficient of the capillary wall

P_c = Hydrostatic pressure within the capillary lumen

Π_c = Oncotic pressure of the plasma

P_i = Hydrostatic pressure of the interstitium

Π_i = Oncotic pressure of the interstitial fluid

The *filtration coefficient (K_f)* of a capillary reflects the intrinsic permeability of the capillary

wall to the movement of fluid, as well as the surface area available for filtration. The K_f can vary between different capillary beds. For example, the K_f of glomerular capillaries is approximately 100 times greater in magnitude than that of skeletal muscle capillaries.

The hydrostatic pressure within the lumen of a capillary (P_c) is a force for the movement of fluid from the lumen into the interstitium. Its magnitude depends upon arterial pressure, venous pressure, and precapillary (arteriolar) and postcapillary (venules and small vein) resistances. In general, an increase in the arterial and venous pressures results in an increase in P_c, while a decrease in these pressures has the opposite effect. P_c also increases with a decrease in precapillary resistance or an increase in postcapillary resistance. Likewise, an increase in precapillary resistance or a decrease in postcapillary resistance decreases P_c. The magnitude of P_c can also vary between tissues, within a given tissue, and is dependent upon the physiological state of the individual. Measurements made in capillaries of the skin, for example, show average values of approximately 32 mm Hg at the arterial end of the capillary and 15 mm Hg at the venous end.

The hydrostatic pressure within the interstitium (P_i) opposes the movement of fluid out of the capillary lumen. This pressure is difficult to measure, but in the absence of edema (abnormal accumulation of fluid in the interstitium), its value is near zero.

The oncotic pressure of plasma proteins (Π_c) retards the movement of fluid out of the capillary lumen. At a normal plasma protein concentration, Π_c has a value of approximately 25 mm Hg.

Small amounts of protein, principally albumin, leak across the capillary wall and enter the interstitium. The oncotic pressure generated by these interstitial proteins (Π_i) promotes the movement of fluid out of the capillary lumen. Typically, Π_i is small and has a value of only a few mm Hg.

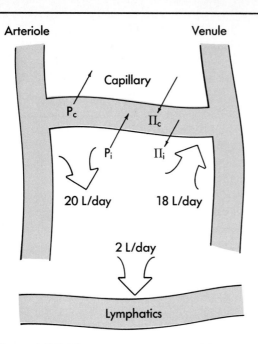

Arteriole   Venule

Capillary

P_c

Π_c

P_i Π_i

20 L/day   18 L/day

2 L/day

Lymphatics

Figure 1-5 ■ Schematic representation of the forces responsible for the filtration and absorption of fluid across the capillary wall. P_c = capillary hydrostatic pressure; P_i = interstitial hydrostatic pressure; Π_c = capillary oncotic pressure; Π_i = interstitial oncotic pressure. For all capillary beds in the body combined (except the glomeruli), approximately 20 L/day is filtered, 18 L/day is absorbed, and 2 L/day is taken up by the lymphatics.

Figure 1-5 is a schematic of the Starling forces across a typical capillary (see Chapter 3 for the glomerular capillaries). As depicted, the balance of forces causes fluid to leave the capillary at the arterial end (filtration) and reenter at the venous end (absorption). Excluding the glomerular capillaries, which filter large volumes of plasma (180 L/day), only about 2% of the plasma flowing through the capillary beds (20 L/day), enters the interstitium. Of this, 18 L/day is absorbed at the venous end, with the remaining 2 L/day returned to circulation via the lymphatic system.

Cellular Fluid Exchange

Osmotic pressure differences between ECF and ICF are responsible for fluid movement between these compartments. Because the plasma membranes of cells are highly permeable to water, a change in the osmolality of either ICF or ECF will result in the rapid movement of water between these compartments. Thus, *except for transient changes, the ICF and ECF compartments are in osmotic equilibrium.*

In contrast to water, the movement of ions across cell membranes is variable and depends on the presence of specific membrane transporters. Consequently, as a first approximation, fluid exchange between ICF and ECF under pathophysiological conditions can be analyzed by assuming that appreciable shifts of ions between the compartments does not occur. This can best be illustrated by considering the consequences of adding water, NaCl, or isotonic saline to the ECF (Figure 1-6).

Example #1—addition of 2 L of water to ECF: When water is added to ECF, the osmolality of this compartment is reduced. If no fluid shifts occurred, the osmolality of the ECF would decrease from 290 to 254 mOsm/kg H_2O. However, the cell membranes are freely permeable to water, and the osmotic gradient resulting from its addition to the compartment will cause water to move into the cells. This water shift will result in increases in the volumes of ICF and ECF above their initial values. The osmolality of the body fluids will also be reduced, but to a lesser degree than that which occurs in the absence of such a shift. Figure 1-6 illustrates the volumes and osmolalities of ICF and ECF after equilibration. These are calculated as follows:

Initial conditions

Initial total body water	= 0.6 × (70 kg) = 42 L
Initial ICF volume	= 0.4 × (70 kg) = 28 L
Initial ECF volume	= 0.2 × (70 kg) = 14 L

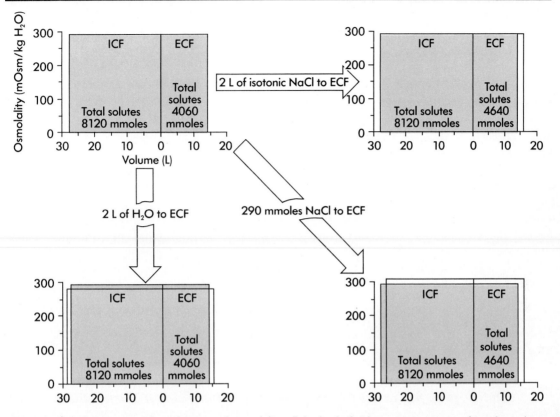

Figure 1-6 ■ Alterations in the volumes and osmolality of the body fluid compartments resulting from the addition to the ECF of 2 L of water, 290 mmoles of NaCl (580 mOsmoles of solute), and 2 L of isotonic saline. The original conditions are indicated by shading.

Initial conditions

Initial total body osmoles =	(Total body water)(Body fluid osmolality)
	= (42 L)(290 mOsm/kg H_2O) = 12,180 mOsm
Initial ICF osmoles	= (ICF volume)(Body fluid osmolality)
	= (28 L)(290 mOsm/kg H_2O) = 8,120 mOsm
Initial ECF osmoles	= Total body osmoles − ICF osmoles
	= 12,180 mOsm − 8,120 mOsm = 4,060 mOsm

Final conditions

Final osmolality	$= \dfrac{\text{Total body osmoles}}{\text{New total body water}} = \dfrac{12{,}180 \text{ mOsm}}{44 \text{ L}} =$ 277 mOsm/kg H_2O
Final ICF volume	$= \dfrac{\text{ICF osmoles}}{\text{New osmolality}} = \dfrac{8{,}120 \text{ mOsm}}{277 \text{ mOsm/kg } H_2O} =$ 29.3 L
Final ECF volume	= New body water − Final ICF volume = 44 L − 29.3 L = 14.7 L

Example #2—addition of 290 mmole NaCl to ECF: $Na^+ - K^+ - ATPase$ in cell membranes restricts NaCl to the ECF space. Because NaCl dissociates into two particles, 580 mOsm will be added to the ECF compartment. Assuming no fluid shift occurs, the osmolality would transiently increase from 290 to 331 mOsm/kg H_2O. However, such an increase in ECF osmolality will result in the movement of water out of the ICF. As a consequence, the ICF volume will be decreased, and the ECF volume will be increased above their initial values. Figure 1-6 illustrates the volumes and osmolalities of ICF and ECF after equilibration. These are calculated as follows:

$$Final\ osmolality\ = \frac{Total\ body\ osmoles}{Total\ body\ water} =$$
$$\frac{12,180\ mOsm\ +\ 580\ mOsm}{42\ L} =$$
$$304\ mOsm/kg\ H_2O$$

$$Final\ ICF\ volume\ = \frac{ICF\ osmoles}{New\ osmolality} =$$
$$\frac{8,120\ osm}{304\ mOsm/kg\ H_2O} = 26.7\ L$$

$$Final\ ECF\ volume = New\ body\ water\ - Final\ ICF\ volume$$
$$= 42\ L\ -\ 26.7\ L\ =\ 15.3\ L$$

Example #3—addition of 2 L of isotonic saline to ECF: The addition of isotonic saline (osmolality = 290 mOsm/kg H_2O) to ECF will not result in a change in the osmolality of this compartment. Consequently, there will be no osmotic force for a fluid shift between the ICF and ECF, and the entire 2 L of isotonic saline will remain in the ECF. Figure 1-6 illustrates the volumes and osmolalities of ICF and ECF after equilibration. These are calculated as follows:

$$Final\ osmolality\ =\ 290\ mOsm/kg\ H_2O\ (Unchanged\ from\ initial\ value)$$

Principles for analysis of fluid shifts between ICF and ECF

- The volumes of the various body fluid compartments can be estimated in the normal adult by the following:

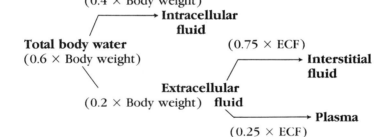

- All exchanges of water and solutes with the external environment occur through ECF (e.g, intravenous infusion and intake or loss via the gastrointestinal tract). Changes in ICF are secondary to fluid shifts between the ECF and ICF. Fluid shifts only occur if the perturbation of the ECF alters its osmolality.
- Except for brief periods of seconds to minutes, the ICF and ECF are in osmotic equilibrium. A measurement of plasma osmolality will provide a measure of both ECF and ICF osmolality.
- For the sake of simplification, it can be assumed that equilibration between the ICF and ECF occurs only by movement of water, and not by movement of osmotically active solutes.
- Conservation of mass must be maintained, especially when considering the addition of water and/or solutes to the body or their excretion from the body.

Final ECF volume = Initial ECF volume + 2 L isotonic
saline = 14 L + 2 L = 16 L

Final ICF volume = 28 L (Unchanged from initial value)

The basic principles and approaches used to examine problems related to the exchange of fluid between ICF and ECF are summarized in the box on page 12.

■ KEY WORDS AND CONCEPTS

- Molarity
- Equivalence
- Osmosis
- Osmotic pressure
- van't Hoff's law
- Osmolarity and osmolality
- Oncotic pressure
- Tonicity (isotonic, hypotonic, and hypertonic)
- Specific gravity
- Effective and ineffective osmoles
- Total body water
- Intracellular fluid
- Extracellular fluid
- Interstitial fluid
- Plasma
- Capillary fluid exchange
- Capillary endothelium
- Starling forces
- Capillary filtration coefficient (K_f)
- Cellular fluid exchange

■ SELF-STUDY PROBLEMS

1. Inulin and tritiated water (THO) are infused intravenously into an individual. The following data are obtained:

	Infusion	Urine excretion	Plasma concentration
Inulin	20 g	12 g	0.5 mg/ml
THO	5 × 10⁶ cpm	2 × 10⁵ cpm	100 cpm/ml

Calculate the following:
   a. Total body water: _____ L
   b. ECF volume: _____ L
   c. ICF volume: _____ L

2. An individual's plasma [Na^+] is measured and found to be 130 mEq/L (normal = 145 mEq/L). What is the individual's estimated plasma osmolality? What effect did the lower than normal plasma [Na^+] have on water movement across cell plasma membranes? Across the capillary endothelium?

3. A 60 kg individual has an episode of gastroenteritis with vomiting and diarrhea. Over a 2-day period, this individual loses 4 kg of body weight. Prior to becoming ill, plasma [Na^+] was 140 mEq/L, and it is unchanged by the illness. Assuming that the entire loss of body weight represents the loss of fluid (a reasonable assumption), estimate the following:

Inital conditions (prior to gastroenteritis)

Total body water:	_____ L
ICF volume:	_____ L
ECF volume:	_____ L
Total body osmoles:	_____ mOsm
ICF osmoles:	_____ mOsm
ECF osmoles:	_____ mOsm

New equilibrium conditions (after gastroenteritis)

Total body water:	_____ L
ICF volume:	_____ L
ECF volume:	_____ L
Total body osmoles:	_____ mOsm
ICF osmoles:	_____ mOsm
ECF osmoles:	_____ mOsm

4. A 50 kg individual with a plasma [Na^+] of 145 mEq/L is infused with 5 g/kg of mannitol (molecular weight of mannitol = 182 g/mole). After equilibration, estimate the following, assuming that mannitol is restricted to the ECF compartment, that no excretion occurs, and that the infusion volume of the mannitol solution is negligible (total body water unchanged):

Initial conditions (prior to gastroenteritis)

Total body water: _____ L
ICF volume: _____ L
ECF volume: _____ L
Total body osmoles: _____ mOsm
ICF osmoles: _____ mOsm
ECF osmoles: _____ mOsm

New equilibrium conditions (after mannitol infusion)

Total body water: _____ L
ICF volume: _____ L
ECF volume: _____ L
Total body osmoles: _____ mOsm
ICF osmoles: _____ mOsm
ECF osmoles: _____ mOsm
Plasma osmolality: _____ mOsm/kg H_2O
Plasma [Na^+]: _____ mEq/L

5. Two normal individuals, each weighing 70 kg with a P_{osm} of 290 mOsm/kg H_2O, excrete the following urine over the same time period:

Individual A: 1 L of urine having an osmolality of 1,200 mOsm/kg H_2O

Individual B: 3 L of urine having an osmolality of 300 mOsm/kg H_2O

If neither individual has any fluid intake, who will have the higher plasma osmolality?

2 Structure and Function of the Kidneys and the Lower Urinary Tract

■ OBJECTIVES

1. Describe the location of the kidneys and their gross anatomical features.
2. Describe the different parts of the nephron and their location within the cortex and medulla.
3. Identify the components of the glomerulus and the cell types located in each component.
4. Describe the structure of glomerular cap-

illaries and identify which structures are filtration barriers to plasma proteins.
5. Describe the components of the juxtaglomerular apparatus and the cells located in each component.
6. Describe the blood supply to the kidneys.
7. Describe the innervation of the kidneys.
8. Describe the anatomy and physiology of the lower urinary tract.

■ STRUCTURE OF THE KIDNEYS

Gross Anatomy

The kidneys are paired organs that lie on the posterior wall of the abdomen behind the peritoneum on either side of the vertebral column. In the adult human, each kidney weighs between 115 to 170 g and is approximately 11 cm in length, 6 cm in width, and 3 cm thick.

The gross anatomical features of the mammalian kidney are depicted in Figure 2-1. The medial side of each kidney contains an indentation through which pass the renal artery and vein, nerves, and pelvis. On the cut surface of a bisected kidney, two regions are evident: an outer region called the *cortex,* and an inner region called the *medulla.* The cortex and me-

dulla are composed of *nephrons,* blood vessels, lymphatics, and nerves.

The medulla in the human kidney is divided into 8 to 18 conical masses, called *renal pyramids.* The base of each pyramid originates at the corticomedullary border, and the apex terminates in the papilla that lies within the *pelvic space.* The *pelvis* is the upper, expanded region of the *ureter,* which carries urine from the pelvic space to the urinary bladder. In the human kidney, the pelvis divides into two or three open-ended pouches, the *major calices,* that extend outward from the dilated end of the pelvis. Each major calix divides into *minor calices,* which collect the urine expressed from each papilla. The walls of the calices, pelvis, and ure-

15

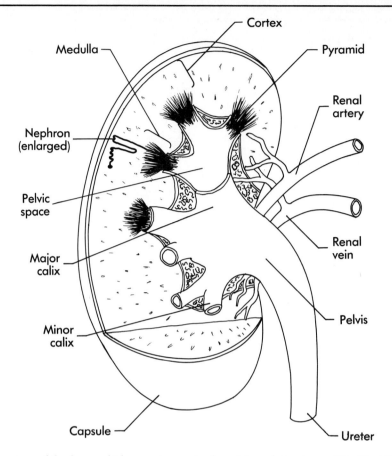

Figure 2-1 ■ Structure of the human kidney, cut open to show internal structures. (Modified from Marsh DJ: Renal physiology, New York, 1983, Raven Press.)

ter contain smooth muscle that contracts to propel the urine toward the *bladder.*

The blood flow to the two kidneys is equal to 25% (1.25 L/min) of the cardiac output in resting subjects. However, the kidneys constitute less than 0.5% of the total body weight. As illustrated in Figure 2-2, *left,* the *renal artery* enters the kidney beside the ureter and branches to progressively form the *interlobar artery,* the *arcuate artery,* the *interlobular artery* (cortical radial artery), and the *afferent arteriole,* which leads into the *glomerular capillaries.*

The glomerular capillaries coalesce to form the *efferent arteriole,* which leads into a second

capillary network, the *peritubular capillaries.* These capillaries supply blood to the nephron. The vessels of the venous system run parallel to the arterial vessels and progressively form the *interlobular vein* (cortical radial vein), the *arcuate vein,* the *interlobar vein,* and the *renal vein,* which courses beside the ureter.

Ultrastructure of the Nephron

The functional unit of the kidney is the nephron. Figure 2-2, *right* illustrates the human nephron. Each human kidney contains approximately 1,200,000 nephrons, which are hollow tubes composed of a single cell layer. The nephron consists of a *renal corpuscle (glomerulus),*

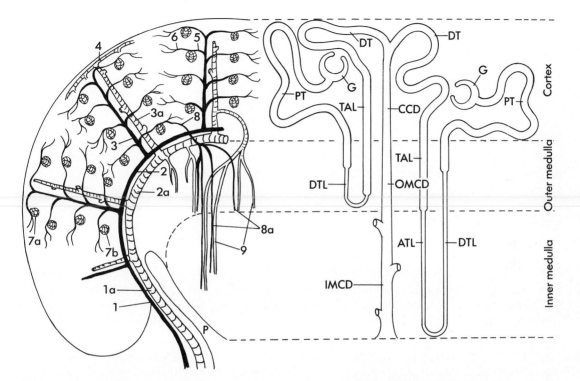

Figure 2-2 ■ **Left Panel,** Organization of the vascular system of the human kidney. This scheme depicts the course and distribution of the intrarenal blood vessels; peritubular capillaries are not shown. (This illustration is not drawn to scale.) The renal artery branches form interlobar arteries *(1)*, which give rise to arcuate arteries *(2)*. Arcuate arteries lead to interlobular arteries *(3)* that ascend toward the renal capsule and branch to form afferent arterioles *(5)*. Afferent arterioles branch to form glomerular capillary networks *(7a,b)*, which then coalesce to form efferent arterioles *(6)*. The efferent arterioles of the outer cortical nephrons form capillary networks (not shown) that suffuse the cells in the cortex. The efferent arterioles of the juxtamedullary nephrons divide into descending vasa recta *(8)*, which form capillary networks that supply blood to the outer and inner medulla *(8a)*. Blood from the peritubular capillaries enters consecutively, the stellate vein *(4)*, interlobular vein *(3a)*, arcuate vein *(2a)* and interlobar vein *(1a)*. Blood from the ascending vasa recta *(9)* enters the arcuate vein. *P*, pelvis. (Modified from Kriz W and Bankir LA: A standard nomenclature for structures of the kidney, Am J Physiol 254:F1, 1988.)

Right Panel, Organization of the human nephron. A superficial nephron is illustrated on the left and a juxtamedullary nephron is illustrated on the right. (This illustration is not drawn to scale.) *DT,* distal tubule; *PT,* proximal tubule; *G,* glomerulus; *CCD,* cortical collecting duct; *TAL,* thick ascending limb; *DTL,* descending thin limb; *OMCD,* outer medullary collecting duct; *ATL,* ascending thin limb; *IMCD,* inner medullary collecting duct. The loop of Henle includes the straight portion of the PT, DTL, ATL, and TAL. (Modified from Kriz W and Bankir LA: A standard nomenclature for structures of the kidney, Am J Physiol 254:F1, 1988.)

a *proximal tubule*, a *Henle's loop*, a *distal tubule*, and a *collecting duct system*.*

The renal glomerulus consists of glomerular capillaries and *Bowman's capsule*. The proximal tubule forms several coils followed by a straight part that descends toward the medulla. The next segment is Henle's loop, comprised of the straight part of the proximal tubule, the descending thin limb (which ends at a hairpin turn), the ascending thin limb (only in nephrons with a long Henle's loop), and the thick ascending limb. Near the end of the thick ascending limb, the nephron passes between the afferent and efferent arterioles supplying its renal corpuscle. This short segment of the thick ascending limb is called the *macula densa*. The distal tubule begins a short distance beyond the macula densa and extends to the point in the cortex at which two or more nephrons join to form a cortical collecting duct. This duct enters the medulla and becomes the outer medullary collecting duct and then the inner medullary collecting duct.

Each nephron segment is composed of cells that are uniquely suited to perform specific transport functions (Figure 2-3). Proximal tubule cells have an extensively amplified apical membrane (the urine side of the cell) called the brush border. This is only present in the proximal tubule. The basolateral membrane (the blood side of the cell) is highly invaginated. These invaginations contain a high density of mitochondria. In contrast, the descending thin limb and ascending thin limb of Henle's loop have poorly developed apical and basolateral surfaces and few mitochondria. The cells of the thick ascending limb and the distal tubule contain abundant mitochondria and extensive infoldings of the basolateral membrane. The collecting duct is composed of principal cells and intercalated cells. Principal cells have a moderately invaginated basolateral membrane and contain few mitochondria, while intercalated cells have a high density of mitochondria. The final segment of the nephron, the inner medullary collecting duct, is comprised of inner medullary collecting duct cells.

Nephrons are subdivided into *superficial* and *juxtamedullary* types (Figure 2-2, *right*). The glomerulus of each superficial nephron is located in the outer region of the cortex (Figure 2-2, *left*, *7a*). Its Henle's loop is short, and its efferent arteriole branches into peritubular capillaries that surround the tubular segments of its own and adjacent nephrons. This capillary network transports oxygen and important nutrients to the tubular segments; delivers substances to the tubules for secretion (i.e., the movement of a substance from the blood into the tubular fluid); and serves as a pathway for the return of reabsorbed water and solutes to the circulatory system. A few species, including man, also possess very short superficial nephrons whose Henle's loops never enter the medulla.

The glomerulus of each juxtamedullary nephron is located in the region of the cortex adjacent to the medulla (Figure 2-2, *left*, *7b*). Juxtamedullary nephrons differ anatomically from superficial nephrons in three significant ways: the glomerulus is larger; the Henle's loop is longer and extends deeper into the medulla; and the efferent arteriole forms not only a network of peritubular capillaries, but also a series of vascular loops called the *vasa recta*.

As illustrated in Figure 2-2, *left*, the vasa recta descend into the medulla, where they form capillary networks that surround the collecting

---

*The structure of the nephron is actually much more complicated; however, for simplicity and clarity, we divide the nephron into five segments. For details on the subdivisions of these segments, consult the references by Kriz and Bankir, Kriz and Kaissling, and Tisher and Madsen (see Additional Reading).

The collecting duct system is not, strictly speaking, part of the nephron. Renal physiologists, however, generally consider it as such. For the sake of simplicity, we will also consider the collecting duct system part of the nephron.

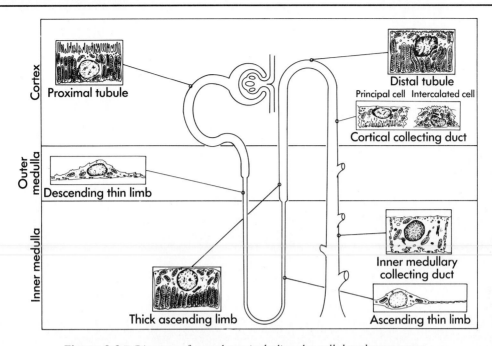

Figure 2-3 ■ Diagram of a nephron including the cellular ultrastructure.

ducts and ascending limbs of Henle's loop. The blood returns to the cortex in the ascending vasa recta. Although less than 0.7% of the renal blood flow enters the vasa recta, these vessels serve important functions. They convey oxygen and important nutrients to the tubular segments, deliver substances to the tubules for secretion, and serve as a pathway for the return of reabsorbed water and solutes to the circulatory system. In addition, as discussed in Chapter 5, the vasa recta are instrumental in the concentration and dilution of urine.

Ultrastructure of the Glomerulus

Urine formation begins with the ultrafiltration of plasma across the glomerular capillaries. *Ultrafiltration* is the passive movement of an essentially protein-free fluid from the glomerular capillaries into Bowman's space. To appreciate the process of ultrafiltration, it is important to

understand the anatomy of the glomerulus (Figure 2-4).

The glomerulus consists of a network of capillaries supplied by the afferent arteriole and drained by the efferent arteriole. During development, the glomerular capillaries press into the closed end of the proximal tubule. The capillaries are covered by epithelial cells called *podocytes,* which form the *visceral layer* of Bowman's capsule. The visceral cells are reflected at the vascular pole to form the *parietal layer* of Bowman's capsule. The space between the visceral and parietal layers is called *Bowman's space.* At the urinary pole of the glomerulus, Bowman's space becomes the lumen of the proximal tubule.

The endothelial cells of glomerular capillaries are covered by a *basement membrane,* which is surrounded by podocytes (Figures 2-4 and 2-5). The capillary endothelium, basement mem-

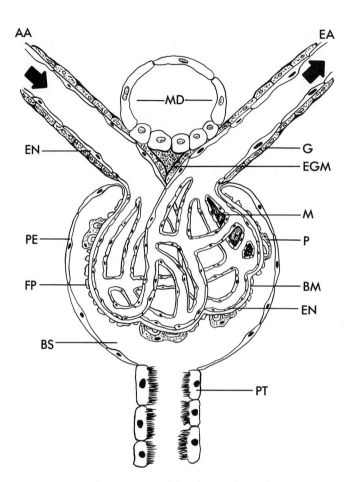

Figure 2-4 ■ Anatomy of the glomerulus and the juxtaglomerular apparatus. *AA,* afferent arteriole; *EA,* efferent arteriole; *G,* granular cells of afferent and efferent arterioles; *MD,* macula densa; *BM,* basement membrane; *FP,* foot processes of podocyte; *P,* podocyte cell body (visceral cell layer); *M,* mesangial cells between capillaries; *EGM,* extraglomerular mesangial cells between the afferent and efferent arterioles; *EN,* endothelial cell; *PT,* proximal tubule cell; *BS,* Bowman's space; *PE,* parietal epithelium. (Modified from Koushanpour E and Kriz W: Renal physiology: principles, structure and function, ed 2, Berlin, 1986, Springer-Verlag Inc.)

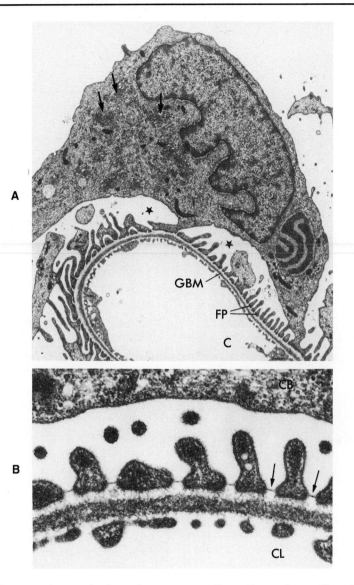

Figure 2-5 ■ **A,** Electron micrograph of a podocyte surrounding a glomerular capillary. The cell body of the podocyte contains a large nucleus with indentations. Cell processes of the podocyte form the interdigitating foot processes *(FP)*. The arrows in the cytoplasm of the podocyte indicate the well-developed Golgi apparatus. *C,* capillary; *GMB,* glomerular basement membrane. Stars indicate Bowman's space. (Magnification ≈5,700x.) **B,** Electron micrograph of the filtration barrier of a glomerular capillary. *CL,* capillary lumen; *CB,* cell body of a podocyte. The filtration barrier is composed of three layers: the endothelium with large pores, the basement membrane, and the foot processes. Note the diaphragm bridging the floor of the filtration slits *(arrows)*. (Magnification ≈42,700x.) (Electron micrographs courtesy of Kriz W and Kaissling B: Structural organization of the mammalian kidney. In Seldin DW and Giebisch G (editors): Chapter 23, The kidney: physiology and pathophysiology, ed 2, New York, 1992, Raven Press. With permission.)

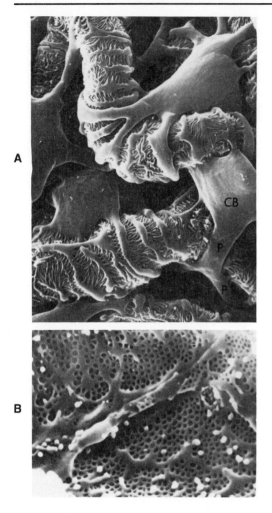

Figure 2-6 ▪ A, Scanning electron micrograph showing the outer surface of glomerular capillaries. This is the view that would be seen from Bowman's space. Processes *(P)* of podocytes run from the cell body *(CB)* toward the capillaries where they ultimately split into foot processes. Interdigitation of the foot processes creates the filtration slits. (Magnification ≈2,500x.) **B,** Scanning electron micrograph of the inner surface (blood side) of a glomerular capillary. The fenestrations of the endothelial cells are seen as small, 70 nm holes. (Magnification ≈12,000x.) (Electron micrographs courtesy of Kriz W and Kaissling B: Structural organization of the kidney. In Seldin DW and Giebisch G (editors): Chapter 23, The kidney: physiology and pathophysiology, ed 2, New York, 1992, Raven Press. With permission.)

brane and foot processes of podocytes form the so-called *filtration barrier* (Figures 2-5, *A* and 2-5, *B*). The endothelium is fenestrated with 700Å (where 1Å = 10^{-10}m) holes and is freely permeable to water, small solutes, such as sodium, urea, and glucose, and even to small protein molecules. Because the fenestrations are relatively large, the endothelium acts as a filtration barrier only to cells.

The basement membrane consists of three layers, the lamina rara interna, lamina densa and lamina rara externa, and is an important filtration barrier to plasma proteins. The podocytes, which are endocytic, have long, finger-like processes that completely encircle the outer surface of the capillaries (Figures 2-5 and 2-6) and interdigitate to cover the basement membrane. The processes are separated by gaps called *filtration slits.* Each filtration slit is bridged by a thin diaphragm that contains pores with dimensions of 40Å by 140Å. As such, the slits retard some proteins and macromolecules that pass through the endothelium and basement membrane. Because the basement membrane and the filtration slits contain negatively charged glycoproteins, molecules are held back on the basis of size, and on the basis of charge. For molecules with an effective molecular radius between 18Å and 36Å, cationic molecules are filtered more readily than anionic molecules (see Chapter 3).

Another important component of the glomerulus is the *mesangium,* which consists of *mesangial cells* and the *mesangial matrix* (Figures 2-4 and 2-7). Mesangial cells surround and provide structural support for the glomerular capillaries; secrete the extracellular matrix; exhibit phagocytic activity; and secrete prostaglandins. Because mesangial cells contract and are located adjacent to glomerular capillaries, they may influence the glomerular filtration rate by regulating blood flow through the capillaries. Mesangial cells located outside the glomerulus (between the afferent and efferent arterioles) are called *extraglomerular mesangial cells* (or

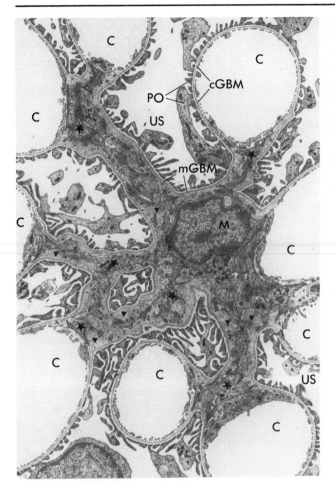

Figure 2-7 ■ Electron micrograph of the central region in the glomerulus showing glomerular capillaries and mesangial cells. The area between capillaries containing mesangial cells is called the mesangium. *C,* glomerular capillaries; *cGBM,* capillary glomerular basement membrane surrounded by foot processes of podocytes (PO) and endothelial cells; *mGBM,* mesangial glomerular basement membrane surrounded by foot processes of podocytes and mesangial cells; *M,* mesangial cell body that gives rise to several processes, some marked by stars; *PO,* podocytes; *US,* urinary space. Note the extensive extracellular matrix surrounding mesangial cells *(marked by triangles).* (Magnification ≈4,100x.) (Electron micrographs courtesy of Kriz W and Kaissling B: Structural organization of the mammalian kidney. In Seldin DW and Giebisch G (editors): Chapter 23, The kidney: physiology and pathophysiology, ed 2, New York, 1992, Raven Press. With permission.)

lacis or *Goormaghtigh's cells*). Lacis cells exhibit endocytic activity.

Ultrastructure of the Juxtaglomerular Apparatus

The structures that compose the juxtaglomerular apparatus are the *macula densa* of the thick ascending limb, the extraglomerular mesangial cells, and the renin-producing *granular cells* of the afferent and efferent arterioles (Figure 2-4). Macula densa cells form a morphologically distinct region of the thick ascending limb that passes through the angle formed by the afferent and efferent arterioles. The cells of the macula densa contact the extraglomerular mesangial cells and the granular cells of the afferent and efferent arterioles. These granular cells are modified smooth muscle cells that manufacture, store, and release *renin.* Renin is involved in the formation of *angiotensin II* and, ultimately, in the secretion of aldosterone. The juxtaglomerular apparatus is one component of an important feedback mechanism that is involved in the autoregulation of renal blood flow and the glomerular filtration rate. Details of this feedback mechanism are discussed in Chapter 3.

Innervation of the Kidney

Renal nerves help regulate renal blood flow, glomerular filtration, and salt and water reabsorption by the nephron. The nerve supply to the kidneys consists of sympathetic nerve fibers that originate mainly from the *celiac plexus.* There is no parasympathetic innervation. *Adrenergic fibers* innervating the kidneys release norepinephrine and dopamine. These fibers lie adjacent to the smooth muscle cells of the major branches of the renal artery, including the arcuate arteries, interlobular arteries, and afferent and efferent arterioles. The renin-producing granular cells of the afferent and efferent arterioles are also innervated by sympathetic nerves. Renin secretion is elicited by increased sympathetic activity. Nerve fibers also innervate the proximal tubule, Henle's loop, distal tubule and collecting duct; activation of these nerves enhances sodium reabsorption by the nephron segments.

■ ANATOMY AND PHYSIOLOGY OF THE LOWER URINARY TRACT

Gross Anatomy and Histology

Once urine leaves the renal calices and pelvis, it flows through the *ureters* and enters the *bladder,* where it is stored (Figure 2-8). The ureters are muscular tubes 30 cm in length. They enter the bladder at its posterior aspect near the base and above the bladder neck. The triangular region of the posterior bladder wall, above the entrance to the posterior urethra and below the point at which the ureters enter the bladder, is called the *trigone.* The bladder is composed of two parts: the *fundus,* or body, which stores urine, and the *neck,* which is funnel-shaped and connects with the *urethra.* The bladder neck, which is 2 to 3 cm in length, is also called the *posterior urethra.* In females, the posterior urethra is the end of the urinary tract and the point at which urine exits the body. In males, urine flows through the posterior urethra into the *anterior urethra,* which extends through the penis. Urine leaves the urethra through the *external meatus.*

The renal calices, pelvis, ureter, and bladder are lined with transitional epithelium composed of several layers of cells: basal columnar cells, intermediate cuboidal cells, and superficial squamous cells. The epithelium is surrounded by a mixture of spiral and longitudinal smooth muscle fibers that are not arranged in discrete layers. The bladder is also lined with transitional epithelium that is surrounded by a mixture of smooth muscle fibers, called *detrusor muscle.* Detrusor muscle fibers are arranged at random and only form layers close to the bladder neck. Here, the fibers form three layers: inner longitudinal, middle circular, and outer longitudinal.

Muscle fibers in the bladder neck form the *internal sphincter.* This is not a true sphincter, but a thickening of the bladder wall formed by converging muscle fibers. The internal sphincter is not under conscious control; its inherent tone prevents emptying of the bladder until appropriate stimuli initiate urination. The urethra passes through the *urogenital diaphragm,* which contains a layer of skeletal muscle called the *external sphincter.* This muscle is under voluntary control and can be used to prevent or interrupt urination, especially in males. In females, the external sphincter is poorly developed; thus, it is less important in voluntary bladder control (see Micturition below).

The smooth muscle cells in the lower urinary tract are electrically coupled, exhibit action potentials, contract when stretched, and respond to parasympathetic neurotransmitters.

The walls of the ureters, bladder, and urethra contain many folds and are therefore highly distensible. In the bladder and urethra, these folds are called *rugae.* As the bladder fills with urine, the rugae flatten out and the volume of the bladder increases with very little change in intravesical pressure. Bladder volume can increase from a minimum of 10 ml following urination to 400 ml with a pressure change of only 5 cm H_2O.

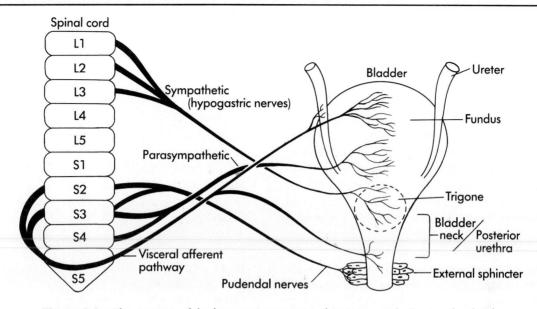

Figure 2-8 ■ The anatomy of the lower urinary tract and its innervation. See text for details.

This illustrates the highly compliant nature of the bladder.

Innervation of the Bladder

Innervation of the bladder and urethra is important in controlling urination. The smooth muscle of the bladder neck receives sympathetic innervation from the hypogastric nerves. *α-adrenergic receptors,* located primarily in the bladder neck and urethra, cause contraction. Stimulation of these receptors facilitates storage of urine by inducing closure of the urethra. *Parasympathetic fibers* via pelvic nerves (muscarinic) innervate the bladder body and cause a sustained bladder contraction. Sensory fibers of the pelvic nerves (visceral afferent pathway) also innervate the fundus. The *pudendal nerves* innervate the skeletal muscle fibers of the external sphincter and cause contraction.

Passage of Urine from the Pelvis to the Bladder

As urine collects in the renal calices, stretching promotes their inherent pacemaker activity.

This initiates a peristaltic contraction beginning in the calices and spreading to the pelvis and along the length of the ureter. This forces urine from the renal pelvis toward the bladder. Transmission of the peristaltic wave is caused by action potentials generated by the pacemaker and passing along the smooth muscle syncytium. The ureters are innervated with sensory nerve fibers (pelvic nerves). When the ureter is blocked with a renal stone, reflex constriction of the ureter around the stone is perceived as pain.

Micturition

Micturition is the act of emptying the urinary bladder. Two processes are involved: the progressive filling of the bladder until the pressure rises to a critical value and a neuronal reflex called the *micturition reflex,* which empties the bladder. The micturition reflex is an automatic spinal cord reflex; however, it can be inhibited or facilitated by centers in the brain stem and the cerebral cortex.

Filling of the bladder stretches the bladder wall and causes it to contract. Contractions result from a reflex initiated by stretch receptors in the bladder. Sensory signals from the bladder fundus enter the spinal cord via pelvic nerves and return directly to the bladder through parasympathetic fibers in the same nerves. Stimulation of parasympathetic fibers causes intense stimulation of the detrusor muscle. Because the smooth muscle in the bladder is a syncytium, stimulation of the detrusor also causes the muscle cells in the bladder neck to contract. Since the muscle fibers of the bladder outlet are oriented both longitudinally and radially, a contracture results in the opening of the bladder neck, allowing urine to flow through the posterior urethra. Voluntary relaxation of the external sphincter via cortical inhibition of the pudendal nerve permits the flow of urine through the external meatus. Voluntary relaxation of the external sphincter is required and may be the event that initiates micturition. Interruption of the hypogastric sympathetic nerves and the pudendal nerves to the lower urinary tract does not alter the micturition reflex. Destruction of the parasympathetic nerves results in complete bladder dysfunction.

■ KEY WORDS AND CONCEPTS

- Cortex
- Nephron
- Pelvis
- Major calices
- Urinary bladder
- Interlobar artery
- Interlobular artery
- Glomerular capillaries
- Peritubular capillaries
- Glomerulus
- Henle's loop
- Collecting duct system
- Bowman's space
- Superficial nephrons
- Vasa recta
- Visceral layer
- Filtration slits

- Filtration barrier
- Mesangial cells
- Extraglomerular mesangial cells
- Juxtaglomerular apparatus
- Detrusor muscle
- Ureter
- Urogenital diaphragm
- Medulla
- Renal pyramid
- Pelvic space
- Minor calices
- Renal artery
- Arcuate artery
- Afferent arteriole
- Efferent arteriole
- Renal corpuscle
- Proximal tubule
- Distal tubule
- Bowman's capsule
- Macula densa
- Juxtamedullary nephrons
- Podocytes
- Parietal layer
- Ultrafiltration
- Mesangium
- Mesangial matrix
- Lacis cells
- Micturition reflex
- Trigone
- Urethra
- Pudendal nerve

■ SELF-STUDY PROBLEMS

1. Review the five major segments of the nephron and the blood supply to the kidney.
2. Review the structure of the glomerular capillaries, basement membrane and filtration slits of the podocytes. Identify the structures that are filtration barriers to plasma proteins.
3. Review the components and structure of the juxtaglomerular apparatus. What is its functional significance?
4. Review the micturition reflex. Discuss the voluntary and involuntary aspects of micturition.

Glomerular Filtration and Renal Blood Flow

1. Describe the concepts of mass balance and clearance, and explain how they are used to analyze renal transport.
2. Define the three general processes by which substances are handled by the kidneys: glomerular filtration, tubular reabsorption, and tubular secretion.
3. Explain the use of inulin and creatinine clearance to measure the glomerular filtration rate.
4. Explain the use of p-aminohippuric acid (PAH) clearance to measure renal plasma flow.
5. Describe the composition of the glomerular ultrafiltrate, and identify which molecules are not filtered by the glomerulus.
6. Explain how the loss of negative charges on the glomerular capillaries results in proteinuria.
7. Describe the Starling forces involved in the formation of the glomerular ultrafiltrate, and explain how changes in each force affect the glomerular filtration rate.
8. Explain how the Starling forces change along the length of the glomerular capillaries.
9. Describe how changes in the renal plasma flow rate influence the glomerular filtration rate.
10. Explain autoregulation of renal blood flow and the glomerular filtration rate, and identify the factors responsible for autoregulation.
11. Identify the major hormones that influence renal blood flow.
12. Explain how and why hormones influence renal blood flow despite autoregulation.

The first step in the formation of urine by the kidneys is the production of an ultrafiltrate of plasma at the glomerulus. The process of glomerular filtration and the regulation of the glomerular filtration rate and renal blood flow are discussed in this chapter. The concept of renal clearance, which enables the measurement of renal function, particularly the rates of glomerular filtration and renal blood flow, is reviewed as background.

■ RENAL CLEARANCE

The amount of a substance in urine reflects the coordinated action of the nephron's various segments and represents three general processes: glomerular filtration; reabsorption of the substance from the tubular fluid back into the blood; and secretion of the substance from the blood into the tubular fluid. These processes are depicted in Figure 3-1, in which the entire nephron population of both kidneys is represented

27

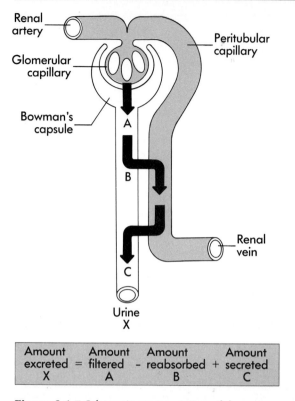

Amount excreted X	=	Amount filtered A	−	Amount reabsorbed B	+	Amount secreted C

Figure 3-1 ■ Schematic representation of the entire nephron population of both kidneys depicting the three general processes that determine and modify the composition of the urine: glomerular filtration **(A),** tubular reabsorption **(B),** and tubular secretion **(C).**

by a single nephron. The concept of *renal clearance* provides an important means for measuring these processes. Renal clearance is based on the principle of *mass balance.* Figure 3-2 illustrates the factors involved in the mass balance relationships of the kidney.

The renal artery is the single input source to the kidney, with the renal vein and ureter constituting the two output routes. Maintaining mass balance, the following relationship can be derived:

$$P^a_x \times RPF^a = (P^v_x \times RPF^v) + (U_x \times \dot{V}) \quad (3\text{-}1)$$

where: P^a_x and P^v_x are the concentrations of substance x in the renal artery and renal vein plasma, respectively; RPF^a and RPF^v are the renal plasma flow rates in the artery and vein, respectively; U_x is the concentration of x in the urine; and $\dot{V}$ is the urine flow rate per minute.

Using this relationship, it is possible to measure the amount of x excreted in the urine vs. the amount returned to systemic circulation in the renal venous blood.

The principle of renal clearance (C_x) emphasizes the excretory function of the kidney in that it considers only the rate at which a substance is excreted into the urine, and not the rate at which it is returned to systemic circulation in the renal vein. Therefore, in terms of mass balance (Equation 3-1), the urinary excretion rate of x ($U_x \times \dot{V}$) is proportional to the plasma concentrtion of x (P^a_x).

$$P^a_x \propto U_x \times \dot{V} \quad (3\text{-}2)$$

To equate the urinary excretion rate of x to its renal arterial plasma concentration, it is necessary to determine the rate at which x is removed from the plasma by the kidneys. This removal rate is the clearance (C_x).

$$P^a_x \times C_x = U_x \times \dot{V} \quad (3\text{-}3)$$

Rearranging Equation 3-3, and assuming that the concentration of x in the renal artery plasma is identical to its concentration in any plasma sample (e.g., arm vein blood sample: P_x), the following relationship is obtained:

$$C_x = \frac{U_x \times \dot{V}}{P_x} \quad (3\text{-}4)$$

Clearance incorporates the dimensions of volume and time, and represents the volume of plasma from which all the substance has been removed and excreted into the urine per unit time. This point is illustrated by the following example:

If a substance is present in the urine at a concentration of 100 mg/ml, and the urine flow rate

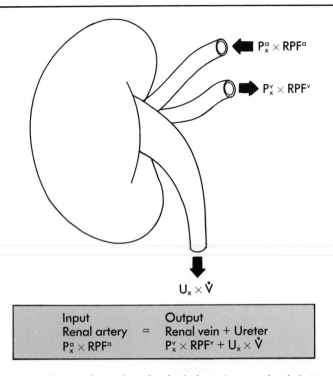

$$P_x^a \times RPF^a$$

$$P_x^v \times RPF^v$$

$$U_x \times \dot{V}$$

Input	Output
Renal artery	=	Renal vein + Ureter
$P_x^a \times RPF^a$		$P_x^v \times RPF^v + U_x \times \dot{V}$

Figure 3-2 ■ Mass balance relationships for the kidney. See text for definition of symbols.

is 1 ml/min, then the excretion rate for this substance is calculated as:

$$\text{Excretion rate} = U_x \times \dot{V} = (100 \text{ mg/ml}) \times \quad (3\text{-}5)$$
$$(1 \text{ ml/min}) = 100 \text{ mg/min}$$

If this substance is present in the plasma at a concentration of 1 mg/ml, its clearance, according to Equation 3-4, is:

$$C_x = \frac{U_x \times \dot{V}}{P_x} = \frac{100 \text{ mg/min}}{1 \text{ mg/ml}} = 100 \text{ ml/min} \quad (3\text{-}6)$$

Measurement of Glomerular Filtration Rate—Clearance of Inulin

Inulin is a polyfructose molecule (molecular weight, ca. 5,000) that can be used to measure glomerular filtration rate (GFR). It is not produced endogenously by the body and therefore must be administered intravenously. Inulin is freely filtered at the glomerulus and is not reab-

sorbed, secreted, or metabolized by the nephron cells. As illustrated in Figure 3-3, the amount of inulin excreted in the urine per minute equals the amount of inulin filtered at the glomerulus each minute:

$$\text{Amount filtered} = \text{amount excreted} \quad (3\text{-}7)$$
$$GFR \times P_{in} = U_{in} \times \dot{V}$$

where: GFR is the *glomerular filtration rate;* P_{in} and U_{in} are the plasma and urine concentrations of inulin, respectively; and $\dot{V}$ is the urine flow rate. If Equation 3-7 is solved for the GFR:

$$GFR = \frac{U_{in} \times \dot{V}}{P_{in}} \quad (3\text{-}8)$$

This equation is the same form as that for clearance (see Equation 3-4). Thus, *the clearance of inulin provides a means for determining the GFR.*

Inulin is not the only substance that can be

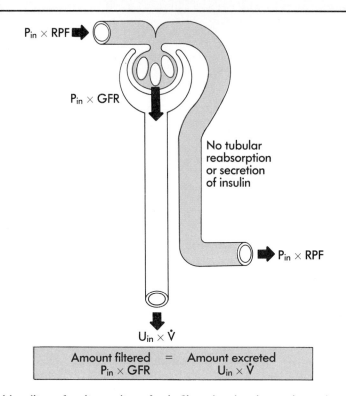

$P_{in} \times RPF$

$P_{in} \times GFR$

No tubular
reabsorption
or secretion
of insulin

$P_{in} \times RPF$

$U_{in} \times \dot{V}$

Amount filtered   =   Amount excreted
$P_{in} \times GFR$ $U_{in} \times \dot{V}$

Figure 3-3 ■ Renal handling of inulin. Inulin is freely filtered at the glomerulus and is neither reabsorbed, secreted, nor metabolized by the nephron. P_{in}, plasma inulin concentration; *RPF*, renal plasma flow; GFR, glomerular filtration rate; U_{in}, urinary concentration of inulin; *V̇*, urine flow rate. Note that all the inulin coming to the kidney in the renal artery does not get filtered at the glomerulus (normally 15% to 20% of plasma, and therefore inulin, is filtered). The portion that is not filtered is returned to the systemic circulation in the renal vein.

used to measure GFR. Any substance that meets the criteria listed in the box on page 31 will serve as an appropriate marker for the measurement of GFR.

While inulin is used extensively in experimental studies, the fact that it must be infused intravenously limits its use in clinical settings. Consequently, *creatinine* is often used to estimate GFR in clinical practice. Creatinine is a by-product of skeletal muscle creatine metabolism. It is endogenously produced at a relatively constant rate, with the amount produced being proportional to muscle mass. Although creatinine need not be intravenously infused, it is not a

perfect substance to measure GFR. Because it is secreted to a small extent by the organic cation secretory system in the proximal tubule (see Chapter 4), an error of approximately 10% is introduced. Thus, the amount of creatinine excreted in the urine exceeds the amount expected from filtration alone by 10%. This is countered by the fact that the method used to measure the plasma creatinine concentration overestimates the true value by 10%. Consequently, the two errors cancel, and the *creatinine clearance* provides a reasonably accurate measure of GFR.

As illustrated in Figure 3-3, not all of the inulin

(or any substance used to measure GFR) entering the kidney in the renal arterial plasma is filtered at the glomerulus. Likewise, not all of the plasma coming into the kidney, and therefore the glomerulus, is filtered.* The portion of plasma that is filtered is termed the *filtration fraction* and is determined as:

$$\text{Filtration fraction} = \frac{\text{GFR}}{\text{RPF}} \qquad (3\text{-}9)$$

where: again, RPF is renal plasma flow.

Under normal conditions, the filtration fraction averages 0.15 to 0.20. This means that only 15% to 20% of the plasma that enters the glomerulus is actually filtered. The remaining 80% to 85% continues through the glomerulus into the peritubular capillaries and is finally returned to systemic circulation in the renal vein.

Filtration Plus Tubular Reabsorption— Clearance of Glucose

Renal glucose excretion is determined by the amount filtered at the glomerulus minus the amount subsequently reabsorbed from tubular fluid by the nephron cells. The amount of glucose filtered at the glomerulus is termed the *filtered load* and is determined by the magnitude of the GFR and the plasma glucose concentration (P_G):

$$\text{Filtered load (glucose)} = \text{GFR} \times P_G \qquad (3\text{-}10)$$

Glucose is reabsorbed from tubular fluid by the cells of the proximal tubule. The transport mechanism for glucose reabsorption is de-

scribed in Chapter 4. For the purposes of this disucssion, it is sufficient to recognize that the glucose transport system can be viewed quantitatively as if it has a maximum transport rate. This is termed the *tubular transport maximum (T_m)*. The T_m for glucose varies from one individual to another, but has an average value of 375 mg/min. Thus, when the filtered load of glucose is less than 375 mg/min, all of the glucose will be reabsorbed and returned to the body via the renal vein. No glucose will appear in the urine, and the clearance of glucose is zero. When the filtered load exceeds 375 mg/min, however, the maximum amount will be reabsorbed into the body via the renal vein; the remainder is excreted in the urine, and some glucose is thereby cleared from the body. Figure 3-4 illustrates these two cases.

It should be apparent from these cases that the renal handling of glucose depends on the plasma glucose concentration. This is illustrated in Figure 3-5, which depicts the relationships between the plasma glucose concentration and its filtered load, excretion rate, and tubular reabsorption rate. As indicated by Equation 3-10, the filtered load for glucose increases linearly as the plasma glucose concentration increases (GFR is constant). Below the T_m, glucose reabsorption is complete, with the reabsorption rate increasing linearly with the filtered load. As a consequence, at these low plasma glucose concentrations, the excretion rate is zero. When the T_m is reached, the reabsorption rate is constant and, in the face of an increasing filtered load, glucose appears in the urine. The plasma glucose concentration at which glucose first appears in the urine is called the *plasma threshold.* Beyond this point, the excretion rate increases linearly and parallels the filtered load.

Careful examination of Figure 3-5 reveals that

---

*Nearly all of the plasma that enters the kidney in the renal artery passes through a glomerulus; approximately 10% does not.

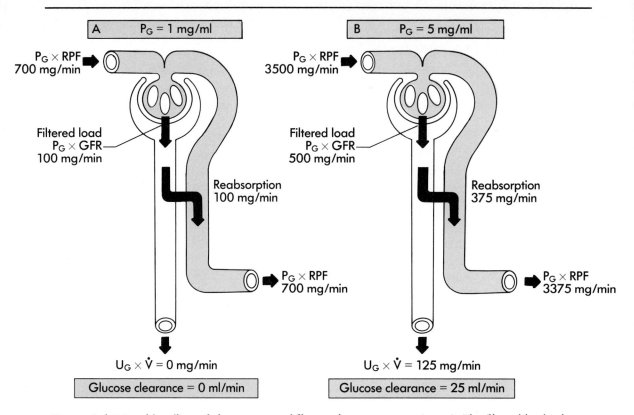

Figure 3-4 ■ Renal handling of glucose at two different plasma concentrations. **A,** The filtered load is less than the tubular maximum (T_m) for glucose. **B,** The filtered load exceeds the T_m for glucose. For both cases the renal plasma flow (*RPF*) is 700 ml/min, the glomerular filtration rate (*GFR*) is 100 ml/min, and the glucose T_m is 375 mg/min. P_G, plasma glucose concentration; U_G, urine glucose concentration; $\dot{V}$, urine flow rate. The clearance of glucose is calculated from equation 3-4.

the reabsorption and excretion curves display a nonlinear transition at the plasma threshold concentration. This "rounding" of the curves is termed *splay.* Splay likely represents heterogeneity in the T_m value for individual nephrons. Thus, although the T_m for the kidneys average 375 mg/min, it may be slightly higher or slightly lower in any given nephron.

Filtration Plus Tubular Secretion— Clearance of PAH

p-Aminohippuric acid (PAH) is an organic acid excreted into the urine by glomerular fil-

tration and tubular secretion. Thus, the amount excreted is the sum of the filtered load and the secreted component. As with inulin, PAH is not produced in the body, and therefore must be infused. PAH is transported by the organic anion secretory system of the proximal tubule, and is further discussed in Chapter 4. For this discussion, it is sufficient to recognize that, like glucose, this PAH secretory mechanism has a transport maximum. Because PAH is secreted from the peritubular capillary into the tubular lumen, it is not the filtered load of PAH that determines whether or not the secretory mechanism is sat-

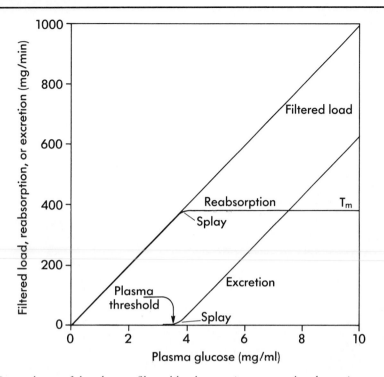

Figure 3-5 ■ Dependence of the glucose filtered load, excretion rate, and reabsorptive transport rate on the plasma glucose concentration. See text for details.

urated. Rather, it is the amount of PAH delivered to the peritubular capillaries.

The T_m for PAH varies from one individual to another, but has an average value of 80 mg/min. Delivery of PAH to the peritubular capillaries at a lower rate results in nearly all of the PAH being secreted into the tubular fluid, such that little PAH remains in the renal vein plasma. When the plasma PAH concentration is increased (generally above 0.12 mg/ml), the delivery of PAH to the peritubular capillaries exceeds 80 mg/min. As a result, 80 mg/min is secreted into the tubule lumen, and the remainder is returned to systemic circulation via the renal vein. These two cases are illustrated in Figure 3-6.

As with glucose, the renal handling of PAH varies as a function of the plasma PAH concentration. Figure 3-7 shows the relationships between the plasma PAH concentration, its filtered load, secretory rate, and excretion rate. At a constant GFR, the filtered load of PAH increases linearly with an increase in plasma PAH concentration. The secretion mechanism saturates between plasma PAH concentrations of 0.1 and 0.2 mg/ml. Below the T_m, nearly all of the PAH entering the kidney is excreted. When the T_m is exceeded, the secretory component is constant, and the excretion rate for PAH increases in parallel with the filtered load. Splay is seen in both the secretion and excretion curves, again reflecting heterogeneity in the value of the T_m among different nephrons.

Measurement of Renal Plasma Flow and Renal Blood Flow

When the plasma PAH concentration is low enough that the T_m of the secretory mechanism is not exceeded (generally at plasma [PAH] be-

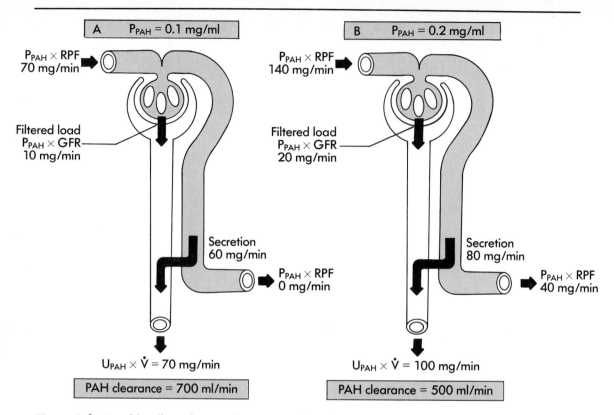

Figure 3-6 ■ Renal handling of p-aminohippuric acid (PAH) at two different plasma concentrations (P_{PAH}). **A,** The P_{PAH} is less than the value that would lead to saturation of the PAH secretory mechanism. **B,** The elevated P_{PAH} results in delivery of PAH to the secretory mechanism exceeding the transport maximum (T_m). For both cases the renal plasma flow *(RPF)* is 700 ml/min, the glomerular filtration rate *(GFR)* is 100 ml/min, and the T_m for PAH is 80 mg/min. U_{PAH}, urine PAH concentration; $\dot{V}$, urine flow rate. The clearance of PAH is calculated from equation 3-4.

low 0.12 mg/ml), its clearance can be used to measure *renal plasma flow (RPF)*.

Figure 3-8 depicts the renal handling of PAH in terms of whole kidney mass balance. It also illustrates why, when nonsaturating (i.e., the T_m for PAH is not exceeded) concentrations of PAH are used, its clearance provides a measure of RPF. The amount of PAH arriving at the kidneys per minute is simply the product of the plasma PAH concentration (P^a_{PAH}) and the RPF. Since all of the PAH is excreted into the urine, and none is returned to systemic circulation via the renal vein, the following mass balance relationship is true:

$$RPF \times P^a_{PAH} = U_{PAH} \times \dot{V} \qquad (3\text{-}11)$$

where: U_{PAH} is urine PAH concentration, and $\dot{V}$ is urine flow rate. Rearranging and solving for RPF, the following equation is obtained:

$$RPF = \frac{U_{PAH} \times \dot{V}}{P^a_{PAH}} \qquad (3\text{-}12)$$

This is the same equation as that for general clearance (Equation 3-4). Thus, at low plasma PAH concentrations, the PAH clearance is equal to the RPF. At high plasma PAH concentrations, however, the PAH secretory mechanism will be saturated, and a significant amount of PAH will appear in the renal venous blood. Under this

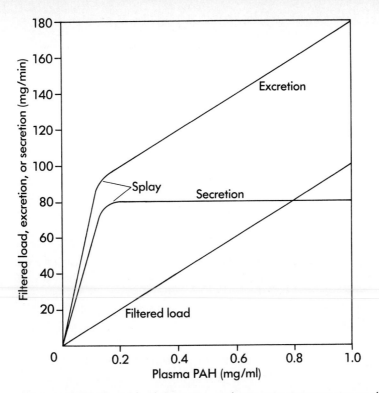

Figure 3-7 ■ Dependence of PAH filtered load, excretion, and secretory transport rate on the plasma PAH concentration. See text for details.

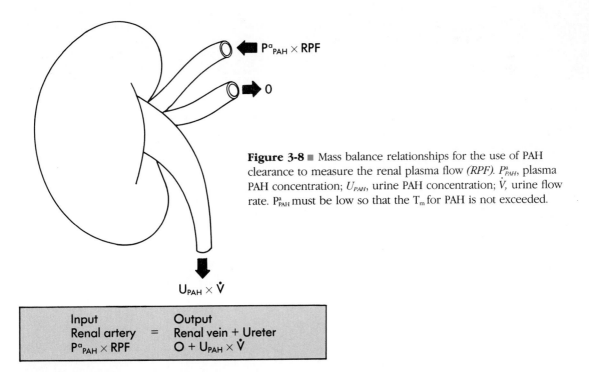

Figure 3-8 ■ Mass balance relationships for the use of PAH clearance to measure the renal plasma flow *(RPF)*. P^a_{PAH}, plasma PAH concentration; U_{PAH}, urine PAH concentration; $\dot{V}$, urine flow rate. P^a_{PAH} must be low so that the T_m for PAH is not exceeded.

condition, Equations 3-11 and 3-12 do not hold; the clearance of PAH does not equal the RPF.

The relationship between PAH clearance and RPF described here is idealized. Even at plasma PAH concentrations that do not exceed the T_m, some PAH still appears in the renal venous blood. The reason for this is related to the anatomy of the nephron and kidney blood vessels. The PAH secretory mechanism is located in the proximal tubule. Consequently, if all of the PAH entering the renal artery were secreted into the tubular fluid, all of the plasma would have to flow through the peritubular capillaries surrounding the proximal tubule. Approximately 90% of plasma does in fact flow through these peritubular capillaries. However, 10% does not; this plasma perfuses some of the medullary structures, the renal capsule, and parts of the renal hilus. Thus, the PAH in this plasma cannot be secreted and is returned to systemic circulation in the renal vein plasma. In recognition of the fact that the clearance of PAH underestimates the true value of RPF by approximately 10%, it is proper to refer to the clearance of PAH as providing a measure of the *effective renal plasma flow (ERPF)*. It is effective in the sense that it represents the plasma flow past portions of the nephron that can effectively secrete PAH.

PAH clearance can also be used to estimate the *renal blood flow (RBF)*. Whole blood consists of a cellular fraction and a plasma fraction. Normally, the plasma accounts for 50% to 60% of the blood volume, and the cells account for the remainder. To determine what fraction of the blood is composed of cells, the *hematocrit (HCT)* is measured. Normally, HCT is in the range of 40% to 50%. Once the hematocrit is known, RBF can be calculated as:

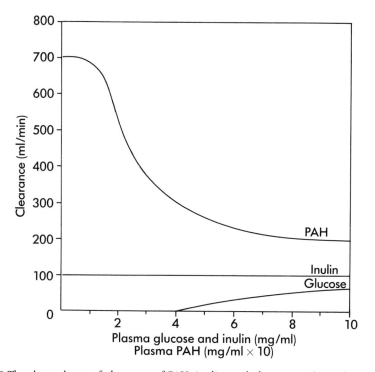

Figure 3-9 ■ The dependency of clearance of PAH, inulin, and glucose on their plasma concentrations.

$$RBF = \frac{RPF}{1 - HCT} \qquad (3\text{-}13)$$

Using Clearance to Estimate Transport Mechanism

As depicted in Figure 3-1, the excretion rate for any substance can be determined as:

Excretion Rate = filtered load − $\qquad$ (3-14)
reabsorption rate + secretion rate

$$U_x \times \dot{V} = GFR \times P_x - R + S$$

Most substances are filtered and either reabsorbed or secreted. The important exceptions to this rule are K^+ and urea, which undergo filtration as well as reabsorption and secretion. If it is known that a substance is filtered freely at the glomerulus, comparison of its clearance to that of inulin (measure of GFR) will indicate net handling of the substance by the kidney. Thus:

1. If its clearance is less than the inulin clearance, the substance is reabsorbed by the nephron (e.g., glucose).
2. If its clearance is greater than the inulin clearance, the substance is secreted (e.g., PAH).
3. If its clearance equals the inulin clearance, the substance is only filtered.

For those substances that are both reabsorbed and secreted, the clearance will reflect the dominant transport system.

It should be apparent that the conclusions about transport mechanism reached from the analysis of clearance values must be considered carefully. Suppose the renal handling of a substance (x) occurs solely by glomerular filtration. If substance x were filtered freely, its clearance would be equal to that of inulin. Now consider what happens when 50% of x is bound to plasma protein. Since only the unbound portion can be filtered and thus excreted, the clearance of substance x will be 50% less than that of inulin. If we did not know in advance that x was partially protein-bound, we would conclude errone-ously that substance x was reabsorbed by the nephron.*

Another point to be made regarding the use of clearance to assess renal function relates to the dependency of clearance on the plasma concentration of the substance. This is illustrated in Figure 3-9, which gives the clearances for inulin, glucose, and PAH as a function of their plasma concentrations. (For all substances and at all plasma concentrations, the GFR is constant at 100 ml/min). Because the GFR is constant, the clearance of inulin is also constant regardless of its plasma concentration (see Equations 3-5 and 3-6). In contrast, the glucose and PAH clearances vary with their plasma concentrations. At low plasma concentrations, the clearance of PAH exceeds that of inulin, whereas the clearance of glucose is zero. As the plasma concentrations of these substances increase, their clearances asymptotically approach that of inulin. The reason for this convergence of PAH and glucose clearances is that, at high plasma concentrations, the secretory (PAH) and reabsorptive (glucose) mechanisms are saturated (T_m is exceeded), and the filtered load becomes a much larger fraction of the total amount of the substance excreted in the urine.

■ GLOMERULAR FILTRATION AND RENAL BLOOD FLOW

The first step in the formation of urine is the production of an ultrafiltrate of the plasma by the glomerulus. The ultrafiltrate is devoid of cellular elements and essentially protein-free. The concentrations of salts and organic molecules, such as glucose and amino acids, are similar in the plasma and ultrafiltrate. Ultrafiltration is driven by Starling forces across the glomerular

---

*When the renal clearance of a protein-bound substance is calculated, the total plasma concentration (bound plus unbound) is used. However, only the unbound portion can be filtered, and only this portion is used to calculate the filtered load (see self-study problems).

Table 3-1 ■ **Relationship between molecular radius and glomerular filterability**

Substance	Molecular weight (g)	Molecular radius (Å)	Filterability
Water	18	1	1
Sodium	23	1.4	1
Urea	60	1.6	1
Glucose	180	3.6	1
Sucrose	342	4.4	1
Inulin	5,500	14.8	0.98
Myoglobin	17,000	19.5	0.75
Egg albumin	43,500	28.5	0.22
Hemoglobin	68,000	32.5	0.03
Serum albumin	69,000	35.5	<0.01

A value of 1 for filterability means it is filtered freely.

capillaries, and changes in these forces and in renal plasma flow alter the glomerular filtration rate. The glomerular filtration rate and renal plasma flow are normally held within very narrow ranges by a phenomenon called autoregulation. This section will review the composition of the glomerular filtrate, the dynamics of its formation, and the relationship between renal plasma flow and glomerular filtration rate. In addition, the factors that contribute to the autoregulation of the glomerular filtration rate and renal blood flow will be discussed.

Determinants of Ultrafiltrate Composition

The unique structure of the glomerular filtration barrier (capillary endothelium, basement membrane and filtration slits of the podocytes) determines the composition of the ultrafiltrate of plasma. *The glomerular filtration barrier filters molecules on the basis of size and electrical charge.* Table 3-1 illustrates the effect of size on filtration. In general, molecules with a radius less than 18 angstroms (Å, where 1 Å = 10^{-10} meters) are filtered freely; molecules larger than 36 Å are not filtered; and molecules between 18 and 36 Å are filtered to various degrees. For example, albumin, an anionic protein that has

an effective molecular radius of 35.5 Å is filtered poorly (approximately 7 g of albumin is filtered each day).* Because albumin is readily reabsorbed by the proximal tubule, however, almost none appears in the urine.

Figure 3-10 illustrates how electrical charge affects the filtration of dextrans by the glomerulus. Dextrans are exogenous polysaccharides that are manufactured in various molecular weights. They take an electrically neutral form, or have negative charges (polyanionic) or positive charges (polycationic). At a constant charge, filtration decreases as the size (i.e., effective molecular radius) increases. For any given molecular radius, cationic molecules are more readily filtered than anionic molecules. The restriction of anionic molecules is due to the presence of negatively charged glycoproteins on the surface of all components of the glomerular filtration barrier. These charged glycoproteins repel similarly charged molecules. Because most plasma proteins are negatively

---

*Approximately 70,000 g/day of albumin passes through the glomeruli. Therefore, the filtration of 7 g/day represents only 0.01%. This is well below the filtration fraction for substances that are freely filtered (15% to 20%).

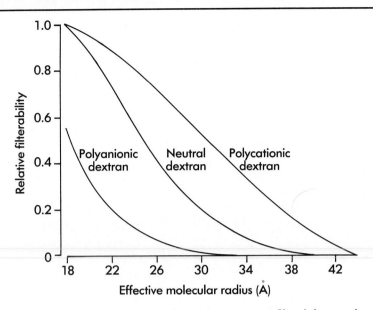

Figure 3-10 ■ Influence of size and electrical charge of dextran on its filterability. A value of one indicates that it is filtered freely, whereas a value of zero indicates that it is not filtered. The filterability of neutral dextrans between approximately 18 Å and 36 Å depends on charge.

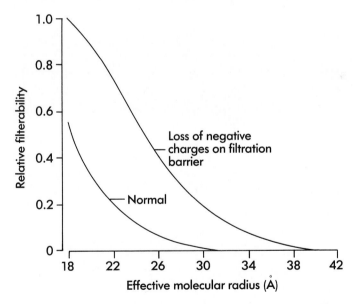

Figure 3-11 ■ Reduction of the negative charges of the glomerular wall results in filtration of proteins on the basis of size only. Injection of antiglomerular basement membrane antibodies into experimental animals reduces the number of fixed anionic charges on the glomerular wall. In this condition, which is known as nephrotoxic serum nephritis, the relative filterability of proteins is dependent only on the molecular radius. In this pathophysiological condition, the excretion of polyanionic proteins (effective molecular radius of 18 to 36 Å) in the urine increases because more proteins of this size are filtered.

charged, the negative charge on the filtration barrier restricts the filtration of proteins.

The importance of the negative charges on the filtration barrier in restricting the filtration of plasma proteins is depicted in Figure 3-11. Removing negative charges from the filtration barrier causes proteins to be filtered solely on the basis of the effective molecular radius. Hence, at a molecular radius between approximately 18 and 36 Å, the filtration of polyanionic proteins will increase compared with the normal state. In a number of glomerular diseases, the negative charge on the filtration barrier is lost. As a result, filtration of proteins is increased, and they appear in the urine *(proteinuria)*.

Dynamics of Ultrafiltration

The forces responsible for the glomerular filtration of plasma are the same as those involved in fluid exchange across all capillary beds. *Ultrafiltration occurs because Starling forces drive fluid from the lumen of glomerular capillaries, across the filtration barrier, and into Bowman's space.* As shown in Figure 3-12, Starling forces across glomerular capillaries are similar to the forces that promote filtration across other capillary beds, and include hydrostatic and oncotic pressures. Both the hydrostatic pressure in the glomerular capillary (P_{GC}) and the oncotic pressure in Bowman's space (π_{BS}) are oriented to promote the movement of fluid from the glomerular capillary into Bowman's

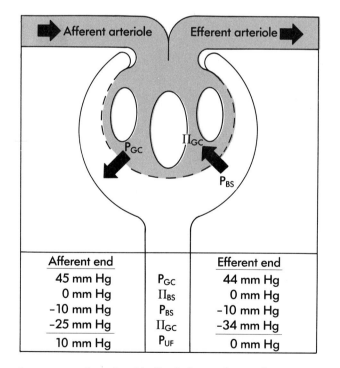

Afferent end		Efferent end
45 mm Hg	P_{GC}	44 mm Hg
0 mm Hg	Π_{BS}	0 mm Hg
-10 mm Hg	P_{BS}	-10 mm Hg
-25 mm Hg	Π_{GC}	-34 mm Hg
10 mm Hg	P_{UF}	0 mm Hg

Figure 3-12 ■ Schematic representation of an idealized glomerular capillary and the Starling forces across the filtration barrier. P_{UF}, net ultrafiltration pressure; P_{GC}, glomerular capillary hydrostatic pressure; P_{BS}, Bowman's space hydrostatic pressure; Π_{GC}, glomerular capillary oncotic pressure; Π_{BS}, Bowman's space oncotic pressure.

space. Because the glomerular ultrafiltrate is essentially protein-free, π_{BS} is near zero. Therefore, P_{GC} is the only force that favors filtration; it is opposed by the hydrostatic pressure in Bowman's space (P_{BS}) and the oncotic pressure in the glomerular capillary (π_{GC}).

As illustrated in Figures 3-12 and 3-13, the net ultrafiltration pressure (P_{UF}) is 10 mm Hg at the afferent end of the glomerulus and zero at the efferent end (where $P_{UF} = P_{GC} - P_{BS} - \pi_{GC}$). Thus, at the efferent end of the glomerulus, filtration equilibrium has been achieved and net ultrafiltration stops. Two additional points concerning Starling forces are clarified in Figure 3-13. First, the hydrostatic pressure within the capillary is nearly constant along its length; the only force that changes appreciably during ultrafiltration is π_{GC}. The increase in π_{GC} results from the filtration of water. Because water is filtered and protein is retained in the glomerular capillary, the protein concentration in the capillary rises and π_{GC} increases.

The glomerular filtration rate (GFR) is proportional to the sum of the Starling forces across the capillaries $[(P_{GC} - P_{BS}) - (\pi_{GC} - \pi_{BS})]$ times the ultrafiltration coefficient (K_f):

$$GFR = K_f\,[(P_{GC} - P_{BS}) - (\pi_{GC} - \pi_{BS})] \quad (3\text{-}15)$$

K_f is the product of the intrinsic permeability of the glomerular capillary and the glomerular surface area available for filtration. Although the P_{UF} is similar in glomerular capillaries and other capillary beds, the rate of glomerular filtration is considerably greater in glomerular capillaries. This is mainly due to the fact that the K_f is approximately 100 times higher; GFR is 180 L/day, whereas net filtration across all the other capillaries in the body is 2 L/day.

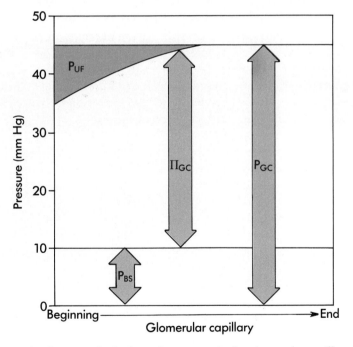

Figure 3-13 ■ Relationship between the hydrostatic pressure in the glomerular capillary *(P_GC)* and Bowman's space *(P_BS)* and the oncotic pressure in the glomerular capillary *(Π_GC)* along the length of an idealized glomerular capillary. P_{UF} is the net ultrafiltration pressure.

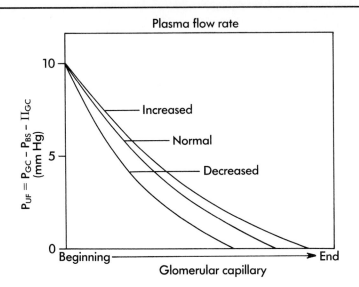

Figure 3-14 ■ Relationship between plasma flow rate along an idealized glomerular capillary and the net ultrafiltration pressure, $P_{UF} = (P_{GC} - P_{BS} - \Pi_{GC})$. Increased plasma flow increases P_{UF} primarily by reducing the increase in Π_{GC} along the glomeruler capillary, and decreased plasma flow decreases P_{UF} by allowing Π_{GC} to increase rapidly along the glomerular capillary.

The second point concerning Starling forces is that plasma flow rate is an important determinant of GFR. Figure 3-14 shows that P_{UF} and GFR are dependent on the plasma flow rate through the glomerular capillaries. As plasma flow rate increases, π_{GC} increases less rapidly, and more filtrate is formed before the capillary oncotic pressure rises sufficiently to stop filtration (i.e., $P_{UF} = 0$). Conversely, if plasma flow rate decreases, π_{GC} increases more rapidly, and less filtrate is formed before the capillary π_{GC} rises sufficiently to stop filtration.

The GFR can be altered by changing K_f or any of the Starling forces. Physiologically, however, there are two primary ways in which GFR is affected:

1. An increase in P_{GC} enhances GFR, and a decrease in P_{GC} depresses GFR. Changes in arterial blood pressure are the most frequent cause of variations in P_{GC}.
2. Variations in renal blood flow affect GFR. As afferent arteriolar plasma flow increases, GFR rises. As plasma flow in the capillaries increases, π_{GC} rises more slowly, and the net ultrafiltration pressure increases. A fall in plasma flow decreases GFR.

Pathological conditions and drugs may also affect GFR, primarily by changing π_{GC}, P_{BS}, and K_f. Thus, GFR may change by three additional mechanisms:

1. Changes in π_{GC}—An inverse relationship exists between π_{GC} and GFR. Alterations in π_{GC} result from changes in protein metabolism outside the kidney.
2. Changes in K_f—Increased K_f enhances GFR, whereas decreased K_f reduces GFR. Some kidney diseases, by reducing the number of filtering glomeruli, reduce K_f. Some drugs that cause vasodilation of the glomerular capillary increase K_f.
3. Changes in P_{BS}—Increased P_{BS} reduces GFR, whereas decreased P_{BS} facilitates GFR. Acute obstruction of the urinary tract (e.g., a renal stone occluding the ureter) increases P_{BS}.

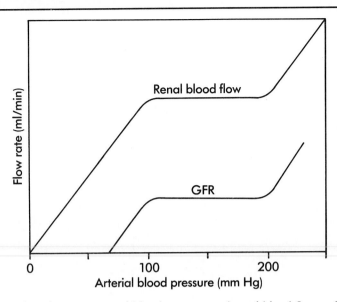

Figure 3-15 ■ Relationships between arterial blood pressure and renal blood flow and glomerular filtration rate *(GFR)*. Autoregulation of blood flow and GFR is maintained as blood pressure changes from 90 to 180 mm Hg.

Renal Blood Flow

The blood flow to the kidneys is equal to 25% (1.25 L/min) of the cardiac output in resting individuals. However, the kidneys constitute less than 0.5% of total body weight. Blood flow through the kidneys serves several important functions, including:

1. Determining the GFR
2. Modifying the rate of solute and water reabsorption by the proximal tubule
3. Participating in the concentration and dilution of urine
4. Delivering oxygen, nutrients, and hormones to the nephron cells and returning carbon dioxide and reabsorbed fluid and solutes to general circulation.

The relationship between GFR and renal blood flow will be discussed below, and the other functions of renal blood flow will be discussed in subsequent chapters.

The equation for blood flow through any organ is:

$$Q = \Delta P/R \qquad (3\text{-}16)$$

where: Q equals blood flow; ΔP equals the difference between mean arterial pressure and venous pressure for that organ; and R equals the resistance to flow through that organ. Accordingly, RBF is equal to the pressure difference between the renal artery and the renal vein divided by the renal vascular resistance:

$$RBF = \frac{\text{aortic pressure} - \text{renal venous pressure}}{\text{renal vascular resistance}} \qquad (3\text{-}17)$$

The afferent arteriole, the efferent arteriole, and the interlobular artery are the major resistance vessels in the kidney and thereby determine renal vascular resistance. The kidneys, like most other organs, regulate their blood flow by adjusting vascular resistance in response to changes in arterial pressure. As illustrated in Figure 3-15, this adjustment is so precise that blood flow remains constant as arterial blood pressure changes between 90 and 180 mm Hg. GFR is

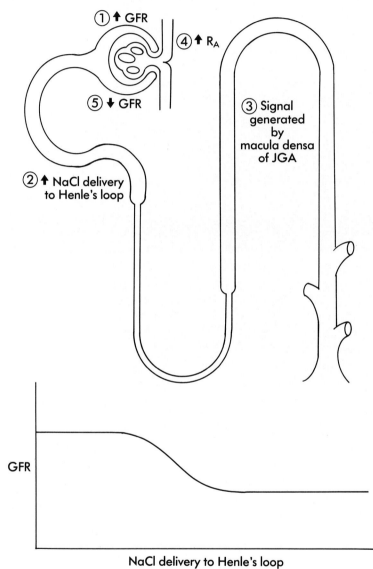

Figure 3-16 ■ Tuboglomerular feedback mechanism. An increase in GFR (1) increases NaCl delivery to Henle's loop (2), which is sensed by the macula densa and converted to a signal (3) that increases R_A (4) which decreases GFR (5). (Adapted from Cogan MG: Fluid and electrolytes: physiology and pathophysiology, Norwalk, Conn, 1991, Appleton & Lange).

also regulated over the same range of arterial pressures. *The phenomenon whereby renal blood flow (RBF) and GFR are maintained constant is called autoregulation.* As the term indicates, autoregulation is achieved by changes exclusively within the kidney. Because GFR and RBF are both regulated over the same range of pressures, and because renal plasma flow (RPF) is an important determinant of GFR, it is not surprising that the same mechanisms regulate both flows.

Two mechanisms are responsible for auto-regulation of RBF and GFR: one that responds to changes in arterial pressure and one that responds to changes in tubular flow rate. The pressure-sensitive mechanism, called the *myogenic mechanism,* is related to the intrinsic tendency of vascular smooth muscle to contract when it is stretched. Accordingly, when arterial pressure rises and the renal affferent arteriole is stretched, the smooth muscle contracts. Because the increase in arteriolar resistance offsets the increase in pressure, blood flow and therefore GFR remain constant (i.e., RBF is constant if the ratio of $\Delta P / \Delta R$ is constant).

The flow-dependent mechanism responsible for autoregulation of GFR and RBF is known as *tubuloglomerular feedback.* As illustrated in Figure 3-16, this mechanism involves a feedback loop in which the flow of tubular fluid (or some other factor, such as the solute composition of tubular fluid) is sensed by the macula densa of the juxtaglomerular apparatus (JGA) and converted into a signal that affects GFR. When GFR increases and causes the flow rate of tubular fluid at the macula densa to rise, the JGA responds and sends a signal that causes RBF and GFR to return to normal levels. In contrast, when GFR and tubular flow rate past the macula densa decrease, the JGA sends a signal that causes RBF and GFR to increase to normal levels. The signal affects RBF and GFR primarily by changing the resistance of the afferent arteriole.

Questions remain about tubuloglomerular feedback concerning the variable that is sensed

at the JGA and the effector substance that alters the resistance of the afferent arteriole. It has been suggested that the macula densa cells sense the osmolality of the tubular fluid or the concentrations of Ca^{++}, Cl^-, or Na^+ in tubular fluid. The effector mechanism may involve the renin-angiotensin system or other vasoactive substances, such as adenosine, prostaglandins, catecholamines, or kinins.

Because mammals engage in many activities that change arterial blood pressure, it is necessary to have mechanisms that keep RBF and GFR constant despite changes in arterial pressure. If RBF and GFR were to rise or fall suddenly in proportion to changes in blood pressure, urinary excretion of fluid and solutes would also change suddenly, because alterations in GFR influence water and solute excretion. Such changes in excretion without comparable alterations in intake would significantly alter fluid and water balance. Accordingly, *autoregulation of GFR and RBF provides an effective means for uncoupling renal function from arterial pressure, and ensures that fluid and solute excretion remain constant.*

Two points concerning autoregulation should be made: Autoregulation is absent below arterial pressures of 90 mm Hg and above arterial pressures of 180 mm Hg, and, despite autoregulation, GFR and RBF can be changed under appropriate conditions by several hormones (see below).

Regulation of Renal Blood Flow

Table 3-2 lists the hormones that have a major effect on RBF. Hormones that cause vasoconstriction, increase vascular resistance, and thereby decrease RBF and GFR include epinephrine, norepinephrine and angiotensin II. Hormones that cause vasodilation, decrease vascular resistance, and thereby increase RBF include the prostaglandins PGE_2 and PGI_2.

Sympathetic Control The afferent and efferent arterioles are innervated by sympathetic neurons that release norepinephrine. Norepinephrine and circulating epinephrine, secreted by the adrenal medulla, cause vasoconstriction by binding to α_1-adrenoceptors on the arterioles and thereby decrease RBF and GFR.

Table 3-2 ■ Hormones regulating renal blood flow

Decrease blood flow	Increase blood flow
Norepinephrine Epinephrine Angiotensin II	Prostaglandins (PGE_2, PGI_2)

Angiotensin II Another major hormone regulating RBF is angiotensin II (see Chapter 6 for details on the renin-angiotensin system). This hormone causes vasoconstriction of the afferent and efferent arterioles and decreases RBF.*

Figure 3-17 illustrates how norepinephrine, epinephrine, and angiotensin II decrease RBF

---

*The efferent arteriole is more sensitive to angiotensin II than the afferent arteriole. Therefore, with low concentrations of angiotensin II, constriction of the efferent arteriole predominates. However, with high concentrations of angiotensin II, constriction of both arterioles occurs.

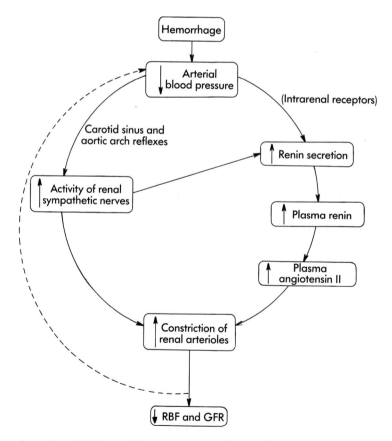

Figure 3-17 ■ Pathway by which hemorrhage activates renal sympathetic nerve activity and stimulates angiotensin II production. See text for details. (Modified from Vander AJ: Renal physiology, ed 2, New York, 1980, McGraw-Hill Inc.)

and GFR during hemorrhage. Hemorrhage causes a fall in arterial blood pressure that activates the sympathetic nerves to the kidneys. Norepinephrine elicits intense vasoconstriction of the afferent and efferent arterioles, thereby decreasing RBF and GFR. The rise in sympathetic activity also increases the production of epinephrine and angiotensin II, which causes further vasoconstriction and a fall in RBF. The rise in the resistance of the kidney and other vascular beds increases total peripheral resistance, which, by increasing blood pressure, offsets the fall in mean arterial blood pressure caused by hemorrhage. Hence, the system preserves arterial pressure at the expense of maintaining a normal RBF and GFR. This exemplifies the point that, although autoregulatory mechanisms can prevent the effects of changes in arterial pressure on RBF and GFR, when needed, sympathetic nerves and angiotensin II have important beneficial effects on RBF and GFR.

Prostaglandins Several prostaglandins, notably PGE_2 and PGI_2, are produced locally within the kidneys and cause vasodilation of the afferent and efferent arterioles. These prostaglandins increase RBF and GFR and tend to dampen the vasoconstrictor effects of sympathetic nerves and angiotensin II, thereby limiting the decrease in RBF and GFR. This is important because it prevents severe and potentially harmful renal vasoconstriction. The stimuli that enhance sympathetic nerve activity and angiotensin II production also increase prostaglandin synthesis (e.g. hemorrhage).

■ KEY WORDS AND CONCEPTS

- Clearance
- Mass balance
- Inulin
- Inulin clearance
- Glomerular filtration rate (GFR)
- Creatinine
- Creatinine clearance
- Filtration fraction
- Filtered load
- Filterability
- Tubular transport maximum (T_m)
- Plasma threshold
- Splay
- p-Aminohippuric acid (PAH)
- PAH clearance
- Renal plasma flow (RPF)
- Effective renal plasma flow (ERPF)
- Hematocrit
- Renal blood flow
- Autoregulation
- Starling forces
- Myogenic mechanism
- Tubuloglomerular feedback
- Hormonal control of RBF (angiotensin II, epinephrine, norepinephrine, and prostaglandins)

■ SELF-STUDY PROBLEMS

1. Pflorizin is a drug that completely inhibits the reabsorption of glucose by the kidneys. The following data are obtained to assess the effect of pflorizin on the clearance of glucose. Fill in the missing data.

   Before pflorizin
Plasma [inulin]:	1 mg/ml
Plasma [glucose]:	1 mg/ml
Inulin excretion rate:	100 mg/min
Glucose excretion rate:	0 mg/min
Inulin clearance:	_____ ml/min
Glucose clearance:	_____ ml/min

   After pflorizin
Plasma [inulin]:	1 mg/ml
Plasma [glucose]:	1 mg/ml
Inulin excretion rate:	100 mg/min
Glucose excretion rate:	_____ mg/min
Inulin clearance:	_____ ml/min
Glucose clearance:	_____ ml/min

   How do you explain the change in glucose excretion and clearance seen with administration of pflorizin?

2. The results of a hypothetical experiment are given on page 48. Determine how substances A, B, C, and D are handled by the kidneys

Substance	Urine [x] (mg/ml)	Plasma [x]* (mg/ml)	$U_x \times \dot{V}$ (mg/min)	Clearance (ml/min)	Filtered load (mg/min)	Transport rate (mg/min)
Inulin	5.5	0.025	———	———	———	———
A	0.8	0.040	———	———	———	———
B	7.5	0.068	———	———	———	———
C	11	0.010	———	———	———	———
D	10	0.060	———	———	———	———

*Plasma [x] represents the total concentration (i.e., bound plus unbound).

(i.e., filtered only, filtered and reabsorbed, or filtered and secreted). It is known that 50% of substance B is bound to plasma protein, and 75% of substance D is bound to plasma protein. Neither substance A nor C are protein-bound. The urine flow rate is 0.5 ml/min.

3. Finding which of the following substances in the urine would indicate damage to the ultrafiltration barrier?
   a. Red blood cells
   b. Glucose
   c. Sodium
   d. Proteins

4. Indicate the Starling forces on the graph below and how they change along the length of the glomerular capillary. How do the Starling forces along the length of glomerular capillaries compare with the Starling forces along muscle capillaries?

5. Describe how an increase in renal blood flow leads to an increase in the glomerular filtration rate.

6. Explain how hormones (sympathetic agonists, angiotensin II and prostaglandins) affect renal blood flow.

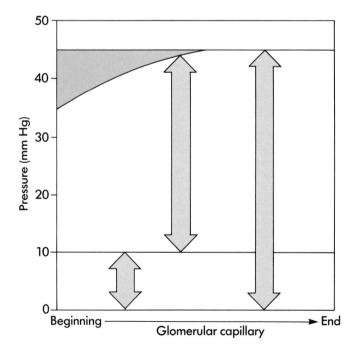

4 Renal Transport Mechanisms: NaCl and Water Reabsorption Along the Nephron

■ OBJECTIVES

1. Explain the three processes involved in the production of urine:
   a. Filtration
   b. Reabsorption
   c. Secretion
2. Describe the magnitude of the processes of filtration and reabsorption by the nephron.
3. Describe the composition of "normal" urine.
4. Explain the basic transport mechanisms present in each nephron segment.
5. Describe how water reabsorption is "coupled" to Na^+ reabsorption in the proximal tubule.
6. Explain how solutes, but not water, are reabsorbed by the thick ascending limb of Henle's loop.
7. Describe how Starling forces regulate solute and water reabsorption across the proximal tubule.
8. Explain glomerulotubular balance and its physiological significance.
9. Identify the major hormones that regulate NaCl and water reabsorption by each nephron segment.

The formation of urine involves three basic processes: ultrafiltration of plasma by the glomerulus, reabsorption of water and solutes from the ultrafiltrate, and secretion of selected solutes into the tubular fluid. Although 180 L of essentially protein-free fluid is filtered by the human glomeruli each day, only 1% to 2% of the water, less than 1% of the filtered Na^+, and variable amounts of the other solutes are excreted in the urine (Table 4-1). Through reabsorption and secretion, the renal tubules regulate the volume and composition of urine (Table 4-2). Consequently, the tubules precisely control the volume, osmolality, composition, and pH of the intracellular and extracellular fluid compartments.

Because of the importance of tubular reabsorption and secretion, the first part of this chapter defines some basic transport mechanisms used by kidney cells to reabsorb and secrete solutes. Then, NaCl and water reabsorption, as well as some of the factors and hormones that

Table 4-1 ▪ Filtration, excretion and reabsorption of water, electrolytes and solutes

Substance	Measure	Filtered	Excreted	Reabsorbed	% Filtered load reabsorbed
Water	L/day	180	1.5	178.5	99.2
Na^+	mEq/day	25,200	150	25,050	99.4
K^+	mEq/day	720	100	620	86.1
Ca^{++}	mEq/day	540	10	530	98.2
HCO_3^-	mEq/day	4,320	2	4,318	99.9+
Cl^-	mEq/day	18,000	150	17,850	99.2
Glucose	mmol/day	800	0.5	799.5	99.9+
Urea	g/day	56	28	28	50

The filtered amount of any substance is calculated by multiplying the concentration of that substance in the ultrafiltrate by the glomerular filtration rate. For example, the filtered load of Na^+ is calculated as: $[Na^+]$ultrafiltrate (140 mEq/L) × glomerular filtration rate (180 L/day) = 25,200 mEq/day.

Table 4-2 ▪ Composition of urine

Substance	Concentration
Na^+	50-130 mEq/L
K^+	20-70 mEq/L
NH_4^+	30-50 mEq/L
Ca^{++}	5-12 mEq/L
Mg^{++}	2-18 mEq/L
Cl^-	50-130 mEq/L
PO_4^{3-}	20-40 mEq/L
Urea	200-400 mM
Creatinine	6-20 mM
pH	5-7
Osmolality	500-800 mOsm/kg H_2O
Glucose*	0
Amino acids*	0
Protein*	0
Blood*	0
Ketones*	0
Leukocytes*	0
Bilirubin*	0

*These values represent average ranges. Asterisks indicate that the presence of these substances in freshly voided urine are measured with dipstick reagent strips. These small plastic strips contain reagents that change color in a semiquantitative manner in the presence of specific compounds. Water excretion ranges between 0.5 and 1.5 L/day. (Table modified from Valtin HV: Renal physiology, ed 2, Boston, 1983, Little, Brown and Company.)

regulate reabsorption, will be discussed. Details on acid-base transport, K^+, Ca^{++}, and PO_4^{3-} transport and their regulation are given in Chapters 7 to 9.

▪ GENERAL PRINCIPLES OF MEMBRANE TRANSPORT

Solutes can be transported across cell membranes by *passive diffusion* or *active transport mechanisms* (see box on page 51). The movement is passive if it develops spontaneously and does not require metabolic energy. Passive transport of solutes, or diffusion, always takes place from an area of higher concentration to an area of lower concentration (i.e., down its chemical concentration gradient). In addition to concentration gradients, the passive diffusion of ions (but not uncharged solutes, such as glucose and urea) is affected by the electrical potential difference, or the electrical gradient, across cell membranes and the renal tubules. Cations, such as Na^+ and K^+, move to the negative side of the membrane, whereas anions, such as Cl^- and HCO_3^-, move to the positive side of the membrane. Diffusion of lipid-soluble substances, such as NH_3, occurs across the lipid bilayer of plasma membranes. Diffusion of water is called osmosis. When water is reabsorbed

Mechanisms of solute transport

Passive

Spontaneous, down an electrochemical gradient, no energy requirement

Diffusion

Facilitated diffusion

Ion channel

Uniport

Coupled transport

Antiport

Symport

Solvent drag

Active

Against an electrochemical gradient, requires direct input of energy

Active transport

Endocytosis

across tubule segments, the solutes dissolved in the water are carried along with it. This process is called *solvent drag* and can account for a substantial amount of solute reabsorption across the proximal tubule.

Facilitated diffusion is a form of diffusion in which transport depends on the interaction of the solute with a specific protein in the membrane that facilitates its movement. Applying this definition broadly, the term facilitated diffusion can describe several different types of membrane transporters. For example, diffusion of ions, such as Na^+ and K^+, through aqueous-filled channels created by proteins that span the plasma membrane is a form of facilitated diffusion. The movement of a single molecule across a membrane by means of a transport protein *(uniport),* as occurs with urea and glucose, is also a form of facilitated diffusion.*

---

*Some physiologists restrict the term facilitated diffusion to this type of transport and use as the classic example the glucose uniporter that brings glucose into a wide variety of cells, such as skeletal muscle cells.

Another form of facilitated diffusion is *coupled transport,* in which the movement of two or more solutes across a membrane depends on their interaction with a specific transport protein. Transport of two or more solutes in the same direction is called *symport (cotransport).* Examples of symport mechanisms in the kidneys include Na^+-glucose, Na^+-amino acid and Na^+-phosphate symporters in the proximal tubule and the $1Na^+,2Cl^-,1K^+$ symporter in the thick ascending limb of Henle's loop.

Coupled transport of two or more solutes in opposite directions is called *antiport (countertransport).* An Na^+-H^+ antiporter in the proximal tubule mediates Na^+ reabsorption and H^+ secretion. With coupled transporters, at least one of the solutes is usually transported against its electrochemical gradient. The energy for this uphill movement is derived from the passive downhill movement of at least one of the other solutes. For example, in the proximal tubule, operation of the Na^+-H^+ antiporter in the apical membrane of the cell results in the movement of H^+ against its electrochemical gradient, out of the cell and into the tubular lumen. This uphill movement of H^+ is driven by the movement of Na^+ from the tubular lumen into the cell down its electrochemical gradient. The uphill movement of H^+ is termed *secondary active transport* to reflect the fact that its movement is not directly coupled with the hydrolysis of ATP (see below). Instead, the energy is derived from the gradient of the other coupled ion (in this example, Na^+).

Transport is active if it depends on energy derived from metabolic processes (i.e., consumes ATP). Active transport of solutes usually takes place from an area of lower concentration to an area of higher concentration. In the kidney, *the most prevalent active transport mechanism is Na^+-K^+-ATPase* (or sodium pump), which is located in the basolateral membrane. Na^+-K^+-ATPase is composed of several proteins that together actively move Na^+ out of the cell and K^+ into the cell. Other active transport mechanisms in the kidneys include H^+-ATPase, which is responsible for H^+ secretion in the collecting duct system (see Chapter 8), and Ca^{++}-ATPase, which is responsible for Ca^{++} movement from the cytoplasm into the blood (see Chapter 9).

Endocytosis is the movement of a substance across the plasma membrane by a process involving the invagination of a piece of membrane until it completely pinches off and forms a vesicle in the cytoplasm. This is an important mechanism for reabsorbing small proteins and macromolecules by the proximal tubule (see the next section for more details). Because endocytosis requires ATP, it is a form of active transport.

In mammals, solute movement occurs by both passive and active mechanisms, whereas all water movement is passive.

■ GENERAL PRINCIPLES OF TRANSEPITHELIAL SOLUTE AND WATER TRANSPORT

The nephron, like other epithelia, such as the intestine, can transport solutes and water from one side of the tubule to the other. *Reabsorption is the net transport of a substance from the tubular lumen into the blood, and secretion is the net transport in the opposite direction.*

As illustrated in Figure 4-1, renal cells are held together by *tight junctions.* Below the tight junctions, the cells are separated by *lateral intercellular spaces.* The tight junctions separate the apical membranes from the basolateral membranes. (An epithelium can be compared to a beverage six-pack: the cans are the cells, and the plastic holder represents the tight junctions.)

In the nephron, a substance can be reabsorbed or secreted across cells, the *transcellular pathway,* or between cells, the *paracellular pathway* (Figure 4-1). Na^+ reabsorption by the proximal tubule is an example of transport by the transcellular pathway. Its reabsorption in this nephron segment is dependent on the operation of Na^+-K^+-ATPase (Figure 4-1). Na^+-K^+-ATPase, which is located exclusively in the basolateral membrane, moves Na^+ out of the cell and into the blood, and moves K^+ into the cell. Thus, the operation of Na^+-K^+-ATPase lowers intracellular Na^+ concentration and increases intracellular K^+ concentration. Because intracellular Na^+ is low (12 mEq/L) and Na^+ concentration in tubular fluid is high (140 mEq/L), Na^+ moves across the apical cell membrane down an electrochemical gradient from the tubular lumen into the cell. Na^+-K^+-ATPase senses the addition of Na^+ to the cell and is stimulated to increase its rate of Na^+ extrusion into the blood, thereby returning intracellular Na^+ to normal levels. Thus, transcellular Na^+ reabsorption by the proximal tubule is a two-step process: movement across the apical membrane into the cell down the electrochemical gradient established by Na^+-K^+-ATPase, and movement across the basolateral membrane against an electrochemical gradient via Na^+-K^+-ATPase.

The reabsorption of calcium (Ca^{++}), magnesium (Mg^{++}) and K^+ across the proximal tubule is an example of paracellular transport. Some of the water reabsorbed across the proximal tubule traverses the paracellular pathway. Some solutes dissolved in this water, Ca^{++}, Mg^{++}, and K^+ in particular, are entrained in the reabsorbed fluid and thereby reabsorbed by solvent drag.

■ NaCl AND WATER REABSORPTION ALONG THE NEPHRON

In the following sections, the NaCl and water transport properties of each nephron segment and its regulation by hormones and other factors are presented.

Proximal Tubule

The proximal tubule reabsorbs approximately 67% of the filtered water, Na^+, Cl^-, K^+, and other solutes (Figure 4-2). In addition,

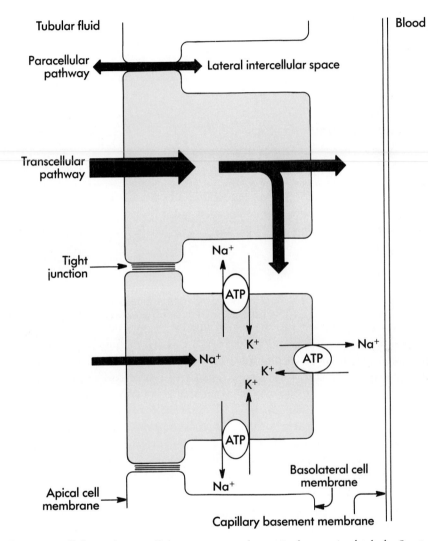

Figure 4-1 ■ Paracellular and transcellular transport pathways in the proximal tubule. See text for details.

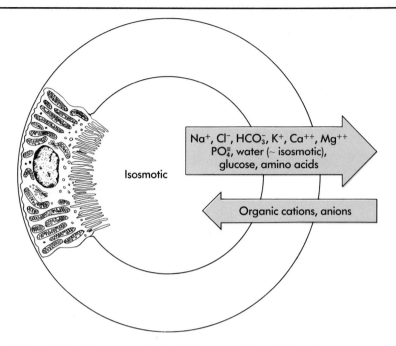

Isosmotic

$Na^+, Cl^-, HCO_3^-, K^+, Ca^{++}, Mg^{++}$
$PO_4^{\equiv}$, water ($\sim$ isosmotic),
glucose, amino acids

Organic cations, anions

Figure 4-2 ■ Tubular profile of the proximal tubule illustrating the cellular ultrastructure and the primary transport characteristics. The proximal tubule reabsorbs 67% of the filtered Na^+, Cl^-, HCO_3^-, K^+, Ca^{++}, PO_4^{3-}, and water and all of the filtered glucose and amino acids. This segment also secretes organic cations and anions. (Modified from Burg MB: Renal handling of Na^+, Cl^-, water, amino acids, and glucose. In Brenner BM and Rector FC Jr (editors): The kidney, ed 2, Philadelphia, 1987, WB Saunders Co.)

nearly all of the glucose and amino acids filtered by the glomerulus are reabsorbed. *The key element in proximal tubule reabsorption is the Na^+-K^+-ATPase in the basolateral membrane. The reabsorption of every substance, including water, is linked to the operation of Na^+-K^+-ATPase.*

NaCl and Water Reabsorption NaCl and water reabsorption by the proximal tubule is divided into two phases: reabsorption of Na^+ with glucose, amino acids, PO_4^{3-}, lactate and HCO_3^- in the first half of the proximal tubule, and reabsorption of Na^+, primarily with Cl^-, in the second half of the proximal tubule. This distinction is based on the types of solute transport systems present in the early and late portions of the proximal tubule, as well as the composition of tubular fluid at these sites. As illus-

trated in Figure 4-3, during the first phase of proximal tubule reabsorption, Na^+ uptake into the cell is coupled predominantly with organic solutes and anions. Na^+ entry into the cell across the apical membrane is mediated by specific symporter and antiporter proteins and not by simple diffusion. Na^+ enters proximal cells by Na^+-glucose, Na^+-amino acid, Na^+-PO_4^{3-}, and Na^+-lactate symporters. Na^+ entry is also coupled with H^+ extrusion from the cell by the Na^+-H^+ antiporter (Figure 4-3). H^+ secretion, via the Na^+-H^+ antiporter, results in HCO_3^- reabsorption (see Chapter 8 for details). The Na^+ that enters the cell across the apical membrane, by either a symport or antiport mechanism, enters the blood via Na^+-K^+-ATPase. The solutes and anions that enter the cell with Na^+ (e.g., glucose, amino acids, PO_4^{3-}, and lactate)

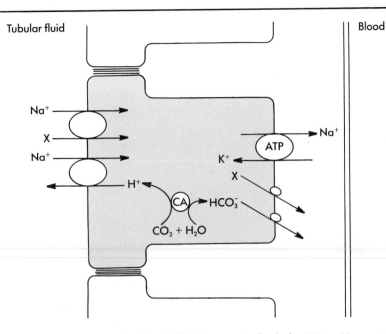

Figure 4-3 ■ Transport processes in the first half of the proximal tubule. $Na^+ - X -$ cotransport protein indicates the presence of five unique symporters. X represents either glucose, amino acids, phosphate, Cl^-, or lactate. CO_2 and H_2O combine inside the cells to form H^+ and HCO_3^- in a reaction facilitated by the enzyme carbonic anhydrase (CA).

exit across the basolateral membrane by passive mechanisms.

In summary, in the first phase of proximal tubular reabsorption, which occurs in the first half of the proximal tubule, reabsorption is coupled with that of HCO_3^-, glucose, amino acids, PO_4^{3-}, and lactate. Reabsorption of glucose, amino acids and lactate is so avid that these solutes are completely removed from the tubular fluid in the first half of the proximal tubule.

In the second phase of proximal tubular reabsorption, which occurs in the second half of the proximal tubule, NaCl is reabsorbed via the transcellular and paracellular pathways. Na^+ is reabsorbed with Cl^- rather than organic anions or HCO_3^- as the accompanying anion. This occurs because the tubular fluid entering the second half of the proximal tubule contains very little glucose and amino acids. In addition, the

tubular fluid has a high concentration of Cl^- (140 mEq/L vs. 105 mEq/L in the first half of the proximal tubule) and a low concentration of HCO_3^- (5 mEq/L vs. 25 mEq/L in the first half of the proximal tubule). The Cl^- concentration is high because Na^+ is preferentially reabsorbed with HCO_3^-, glucose, and organic anions in the first half of the proximal tubule, leaving behind a solution that becomes enriched in Cl^-.

As illustrated in Figure 4-4, paracellular NaCl reabsorption occurs because the rise in $[Cl^-]$ in the tubular fluid creates a gradient that favors the diffusion of Cl^- from the tubular lumen, across the tight junctions and into the lateral intercellular space. Movement of the negatively charged Cl^- generates a positive transepithelial voltage (tubular fluid positive relative to the blood), which causes the diffusion of positively charged Na^+ out of the tubular fluid, across the tight junc-

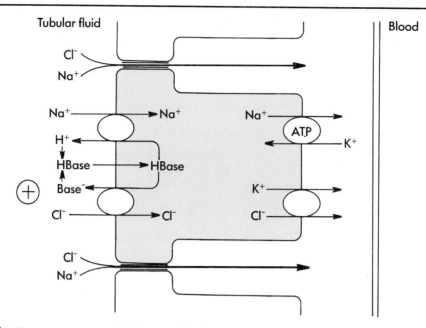

Figure 4-4 ■ Transport processes in the second half of the proximal tubule. Na^+ and Cl^- enter the cell across the apical membrane by the operation of parallel $Na^+ - H^+$ and $Cl^- - Base^-$ antiporters. Because the secreted H^+ and $Base^-$ combine in the tubular fluid to form HBase, which reenters the cell, the net result is NaCl uptake. Base may be OH^-, formate (HCO_2^-), oxalate$^-$, or HCO_3^-. The lumen positive transepithelial voltage is generated by the diffusion of Cl^- (lumen-to-blood) across the tight junction.

tion and into the blood. Thus, in the second half of the proximal tubule, some Na^+ and Cl^- is reabsorbed across the tight junctions by passive diffusion.

NaCl reabsorption by the second half of the proximal tubule also occurs by a transcellular route. As illustrated in Figure 4-4, NaCl enters the cell across the luminal membrane by the parallel operation of Na^+-H^+ and Cl^--$Base^-$ antiporters. Because the secreted H^+ and $Base^-$ combine in the tubular fluid and reenter the cell by passive diffusion, operation of the Na^+/H^+ and $Cl^-/Base^-$ antiporters is equivalent to NaCl uptake from tubular fluid into the cell. Na^+ leaves the cell by Na^+-K^+-ATPase, and Cl^- leaves the cell and enters the blood by a KCl symport protein.

In summary, proximal tubule reabsorption of Na^+ and Cl^- occurs across the paracellular and transcellular pathways. Approximately 17,000 mEq of the 25,200 mEq of sodium filtered each day is reabsorbed in the proximal tubule ($\sim$ 67% of the filtered load). Of this, two thirds moves across the transcellular pathway, and one third moves across the paracellular pathway.

Figure 4-5 illustrates the mechanism of water reabsorption by the proximal tubule. The reabsorption of Na^+ with organic solutes and Cl^- increases the osmolality of the lateral intercellular space. This occurs because some Na^+-K^+-ATPase pumps and organic solute and Cl^- transporters are located on the lateral cell membranes, which deposit the solutes in this space. Furthermore, some NaCl enters the lateral intercellular space by diffusion across the tight junction. Because the lateral intercellular space becomes slightly hyperosmotic (3 to 5 mOsm/kg H_2O) with respect to tubular fluid, and be-

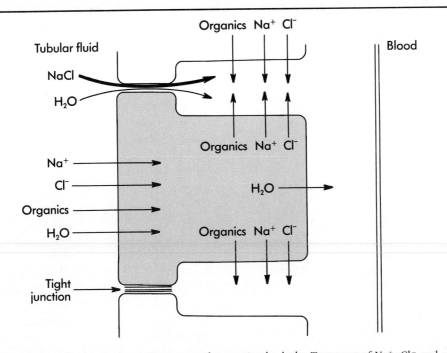

Figure 4-5 ■ Routes of water reabsorption across the proximal tubule. Transport of Na^+, Cl^- and organic solutes into the lateral intercellular space increases the osmolality of this compartment, which establishes the driving force for osmotic water reabsorption across the proximal tubule. Water flows across the paracellular and cellular pathways.

cause the proximal tubule is highly permeable to water, water will flow by osmosis across both the tight junctions and the proximal tubular cells into this hyperosmotic compartment.

Accumulation of fluid and solutes within the lateral intercellular space increases the hydrostatic pressure in this compartment, which forces fluid and these solutes into the capillaries. Thus, *water reabsorption follows solute transport in the proximal tubule.* The reabsorbed fluid is essentially *isosmotic* to plasma. (The osmolality of the reabsorbed fluid is slightly hyperosmotic to plasma; however, for the sake of simplicity, we will consider the fluid to be isosmotic.) An important consequence of osmotic water flow across the proximal tubule is that some solutes, especially K^+, Ca^{++}, and Mg^{++}, are entrained in the reabsorbed fluid and thereby reabsorbed by solvent drag.

Because the reabsorption of nearly all organic solutes, Cl^-, other ions, and water are coupled with Na^+ reabsorption, changes in Na^+ reabsorption influence the reabsorption of water and other solutes by the proximal tubule.

Organic Anion and Organic Cation Secretion In addition to reabsorbing solutes and water, the proximal tubule also secretes organic cations and anions (see Tables 4-3 and 4-4 for a partial listing). Many of these substances are end products of metabolism that circulate in the plasma. The proximal tubule also secretes numerous exogenous organic compounds, including p-aminohippurate (PAH) and drugs such as penicillin. Because many of these organic compounds can be bound to plasma proteins, they are not readily filtered. Therefore, excretion by filtration alone eliminates only a

Table 4-3 ■ Some organic anions secreted by the proximal tubule

Endogenous anions	Drugs
cAMP	Acetazolamide
Bile salts	Chlorothiazide
Hippurates (PAH)	Furosemide
Oxalate	Penicillin
Prostaglandins	Probenecid
Urate	Salicylate (aspirin)
	Hydrochlorothiazide
	Bumetanide

Table 4-4 ■ Some organic cations secreted by the proximal tubule

Endogenous cations	Drugs
Creatinine	Atropine
Dopamine	Isoproterenol
Epinephrine	Cimetidine
Norepinephrine	Morphine
	Quinine
	Amiloride

small portion of these potentially toxic substances from the body. High excretion rates of these organic compounds are obtained by secretion from the peritubular capillaries into the tubular fluid. Because the kidneys remove nearly all organic ions and drugs from the plasma that enter the kidneys, it is evident that these secretory mechanisms are extremely powerful and serve a vital function by eliminating these substances.

Figure 4-6 shows the mechanism of PAH transport across the proximal tubule as an example of organic anion secretion. This secretory pathway has a T_m, a low specificity, and is responsible for the secretion of all organic anions listed in Table 4-3. Information about this pathway has been obtained using the organic anion PAH, which, as described in Chapter 3, can be used

to measure RPF. PAH is taken up into the cell across the basolateral membrane against its chemical gradient by a PAH-dicarboxylate and tricarboxylate antiport mechanism. The dicarboxylates and tricarboxylates accumulate inside the cell via an Na^+-dicarboxylate and tricarboxylate symporter in the basolateral membrane. Thus, PAH uptake into the cell against its chemical gradient is coupled with movement of dicarboxylates and tricarboxylates down their chemical gradients via the antiport mechanism. The resulting high concentration of PAH in the cell provides the driving force for PAH to exit across the luminal membrane into the tubular fluid via a PAH-anion antiporter. Because there is competition for transport among all organic anions, elevated plasma levels of one anion inhibits the secretion of the others. For example, a reduction of penicillin secretion can be produced by infusing PAH.

The active secretory pathway for organic cations in the proximal tubule is analogous to that of organic anions, although the precise details of the mechanism have not been explained. The pathway for organic cations is nonspecific (see Table 4-4) and has a T_m, with several organic cations competing for transport.

Protein Reabsorption The proximal tubule also reabsorbs proteins. As discussed in Chapter 3, peptide hormones, small proteins, and even small amounts of larger proteins, such as albumin, are filtered by the glomerulus. Although protein filtration is small (the concentration of proteins in the ultrafiltrate is only 40 mg/L), the amount of protein filtered per day is significant (filtered protein = GFR × [protein] in the ultrafiltrate; thus, filtered protein = 180 L/day × 40 mg/L = 7.2 g/day) because the GFR is so high. These proteins are partially degraded by enzymes on the surface of the proximal tubule cells and taken up into the cell by endocytosis. Once inside the cell, the endocytic vesicles fuse with lysosomes, which contain enzymes that digest the proteins and peptides into their constituent amino acids. The amino acids

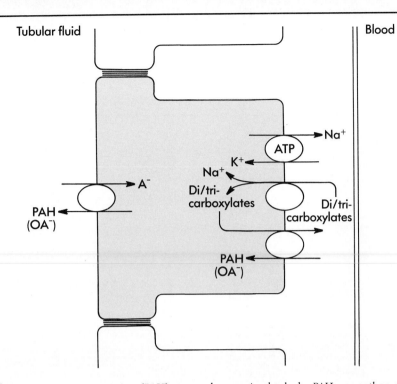

Figure 4-6 ■ Organic anion secretion (PAH) across the proximal tubule. PAH or another organic anion (OA^-) enters the cell across the basolateral membrane by a PAH-di-and tricarboxylate antiport mechanism. The uptake of di-carboxylates and tricarboxylates into cell, against their chemical gradients, is driven by the movement of Na^+ into the cell. The di-carboxylates and tricarboxylates recycle across the basolateral membrane. PAH leaves the cell across the apical membrane, down its chemical gradient, by a PAH-organic anion (OA^-) antiport mechanism. The OA^- indicates one of several possible anions (e.g., urate).

leave the cell across the basolateral membrane and return to the blood. Normally, this mechanism reabsorbs nearly all of the protein filtered, and the urine is essentially protein-free. However, because the mechanism is easily saturated, if the amount of protein filtered increases, protein will appear in the urine. Disruption of the glomerular barrier to proteins will increase the filtration of proteins and result in *proteinuria* (appearance of protein in the urine).

Henle's Loop

Henle's loop reabsorbs approximately 20% of the filtered Na^+, Cl^-, and K^+ (Figure 4-7). Ca^{++}, HCO_3^-, and Mg^{++} are also reabsorbed here (see Chapters 7 through 9). This reabsorption occurs almost exclusively in the thick ascending limb. By comparison, the ascending thin limb has a much lower reabsorptive capacity, and the descending thin limb does not reabsorb significant amounts of solutes (see Chapter 5).

Henle's loop reabsorbs approximately 20% of the filtered water. This reabsorption, however, occurs exclusively in the descending thin limb. *The ascending limb is impermeable to water.*

The key element in solute reabsorption by the thick ascending limb is the Na^+-K^+-ATPase in the basolateral membrane (Figure 4-8). As with reabsorption in the proximal tubule, the reabsorption of every substance by the thick ascending limb is linked to Na^+-K^+-ATPase. Na^+-K^+-ATPase in the thick ascending limb

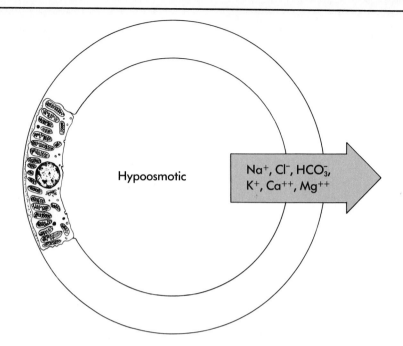

Hypoosmotic

$Na^+, Cl^-, HCO_3^-,$
K^+, Ca^{++}, Mg^{++}

Figure 4-7 ■ Tubular profile of the thick ascending limb of Henle's loop illustrating the cellular ultrastructure and the primary transport characteristics. The thick ascending limb reabsorbs 20% of the filtered Na^+, Cl^-, HCO_3^-, K^+, Ca^{++} and 80% of the filtered Mg^{++}. (Modified from Burg MB: Renal handling of Na^+, Cl^-, water, amino acids, and glucose. In Brenner BM and Rector FC Jr (editors): The kidney, ed 2, Philadelphia, 1987, WB Saunders Co.)

maintains a low cell $[Na^+]$, which provides a favorable chemical gradient for the movement of Na^+ from the tubular fluid into the cell. The movement of Na^+ across the apical membrane into the cell is mediated by the $1Na^+,2Cl^-,1K^+$ symporter, which couples the movement of $1Na^+$ with $2Cl^-$ and $1K^+$. This symport protein uses the potential energy released by the downhill movement of Na^+ and Cl^- to drive the uphill movement of K^+ into the cell. Inhibition of this symporter by loop diuretics, such as furosemide, completely inhibits Na^+ and Cl^- reabsorption by the thick ascending limb.

An Na^+-H^+ antiporter in the apical cell membrane also mediates Na^+ reabsorption and H^+ secretion (HCO_3^- reabsorption) in the thick ascending limb (Figure 4-8). Na^+ leaves the cell across the basolateral membrane via Na^+-K^+-ATPase, and K^+, Cl^-, and HCO_3^- leave the cell across the basolateral membrane via separate pathways.

The voltage across the thick ascending limb is positive in the tubular fluid relative to the blood because of the unique permeability characteristics of this tubular segment. Specifically, the movement of K^+ out of the cell across the apical membrane via a K^+ channel generates a lumen-positive voltage. The magnitude of this voltage varies directly with the rate of K^+ exit from the cell, which in turn varies with the rate of its uptake into the cell by the apical membrane $1Na^+,2Cl^-,1K^+$ symporter (i.e., some K^+ recycles across the apical membrane). It is important to recognize that increased transport by

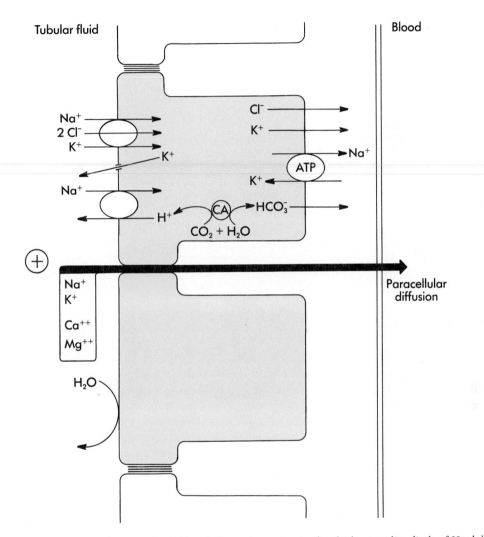

Figure 4-8 ■ Transport mechanisms for Na$^+$ and Cl$^-$ reabsorption in the thick ascending limb of Henle's loop. The lumen positive transepithelial voltage results from the diffusion of K$^+$ from the cell into the tubular fluid, and plays a major role in driving passive paracellular reabsorption of cations.

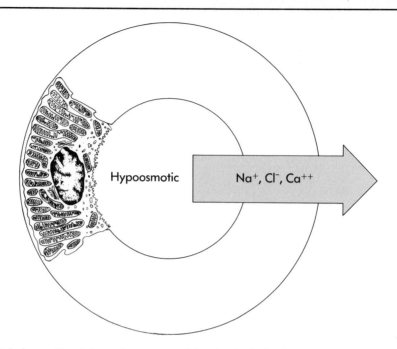

Figure 4-9 ■ Tubular profile of the early segment of the distal tubule illustrating the cellular ultrastructure and the primary transport characteristics. This segment reabsorbs Na^+, Cl^- and Ca^{++}, but is impermeable to water. (Modified from Burg MB: Renal handling of Na^+, Cl^-, water, amino acids, and glucose. In Brenner BM and Rector FC Jr (editors): The kidney, ed 2, Philadelphia, 1987, WB Saunders Co.)

the thick ascending limb results in an increase in the magnitude of the lumen-positive voltage, and that this voltage is an important force for the reabsorption of several cations, including Na^+, K^+, Ca^{++}, and Mg^{++} across the paracellular pathway. Thus, salt reabsorption across the thick ascending limb occurs by two routes: the transcellular and paracellular pathways. Fifty percent of transport is transcellular, and 50% is paracellular.

Because the thick ascending limb is impermeable to water, reabsorption of sodium, chloride, and other solutes reduces the osmolality of tubular fluid to less than 150 mOsm/Kg H_2O.

Distal Tubule and Collecting Duct

The distal tubule and collecting duct reabsorb approximately 12% of the filtered Na^+ and Cl^-, secrete variable amounts of K^+ and H^+, and reabsorb a variable amount of water. The first segment of the distal tubule (early distal tubule) reabsorbs Na^+, Cl^-, and Ca^{++}. Like the thick ascending limb, it is impermeable to water (Figure 4-9). The entry of Na^+ and Cl^- into the cell across the apical membrane is mediated by a NaCl symporter (Figure 4-10). Na^+ leaves the cell via Na^+-K^+-ATPase, and Cl^- leaves the cell by diffusion via channels. Thus, *the early segment of the distal tubule continues the active dilution of tubular fluid that began in the thick ascending limb.*

The last segment of the distal tubule (late distal tubule) and the collecting duct are composed of two cell types, *principal cells* and *intercalated cells.* As illustrated in Figure 4-11, principal cells reabsorb Na^+ and water, and se-

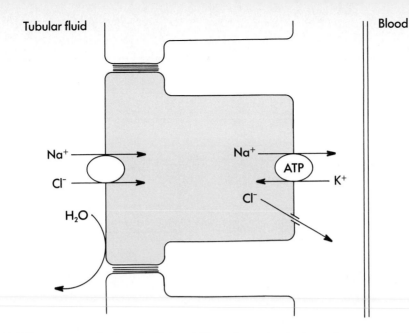

Figure 4-10 ■ Transport mechanism for Na$^+$ and Cl$^-$ reabsorption in the early segment of the distal tubule. See the text for details.

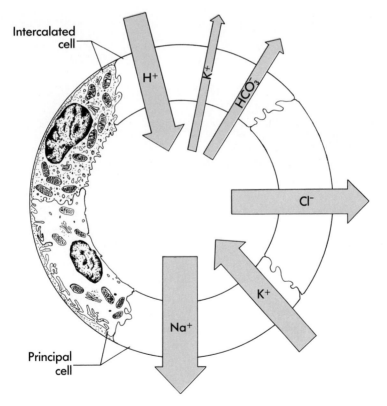

Figure 4-11 ■ Tubular profile of last segment of the distal tubule and the collecting duct illustrating the cellular ultrastructure and the primary transport characteristics. Intercalated cells secrete H$^+$ and reabsorb HCO$_3^-$ and K$^+$, whereas principal cells secrete K$^+$ and reabsorb Na$^+$ and water. The mechanism of Cl$^-$ reabsorption and the pathway are not completely understood. (Modified from Burg MB: Renal handling of Na$^+$, Cl$^-$, water, amino acids, and glucose. In Brenner BM and Rector FC Jr (editors): The kidney, ed 2, Philadelphia, 1987, WB Saunders Co.)

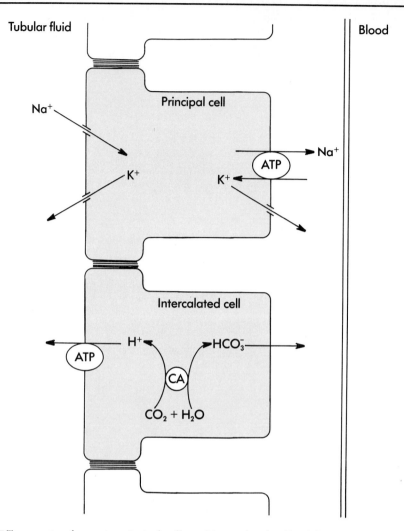

Figure 4-12 ■ Transport pathways in principal cells and intercalated cells of the distal tubule and collecting duct. See the text for details.

crete K^+. Intercalated cells secrete H^+ (reabsorb HCO_3^-) and thus are important in regulating acid-base balance (see Chapter 8). Intercalated cells also reabsorb K^+. Both Na^+ reabsorption and K^+ secretion by principal cells depend on the activity of Na^+-K^+-ATPase in the basolateral membrane (Figure 4-12). This enzyme maintains a low cell $[Na^+]$, which provides a favorable chemical gradient for the movement of Na^+ from the tubular fluid into the cell. Be-

cause Na^+ enters the cell across the apical membrane by diffusion through water-filled channels, the negative potential inside the cell facilitates Na^+ entry. Na^+ leaves the cell across the basolateral membrane and enters the blood via Na^+-K^+-ATPase. Although the collecting duct reabsorbs significant amounts of Cl^-, its mechanism and route of transport are not completely understood.

K^+ is secreted by principal cells from blood

into the tubular fluid in two steps (Figure 4-12). K^+ uptake across the basolateral membrane is mediated by Na^+-K^+-ATPase. Because the $[K^+]$ inside the cells is high (140 mEq/L) and the $[K^+]$ in tubular fluid is low ($\sim$10 mEq/L), this ion will diffuse down its concentration gradient, across the apical cell membrane and into the tubular fluid. Although the negative potential inside the cells tends to retain K^+, the combined electrochemical gradient across the apical membrane favors K^+ secretion from the cell into the tubular fluid. Additional details of K^+ secretion and its regulation are covered in Chapter 7.

Intercalated cells secrete H^+ and reabsorb HCO_3^- and K^+. H^+ secretion across the apical membrane is against an electrochemical gradient and is mediated by an H^+-ATPase transport mechanism (Figure 4-12). The generation of H^+ inside the cell is facilitated by the enzyme carbonic anhydrase and results in the production of HCO_3^-. For each H^+ secreted into the tubular fluid, one HCO_3^- leaves the cell across the basolateral membrane. H^+ secretion and HCO_3^- reabsorption by the collecting duct are further discussed in Chapter 8. The mechanism of K^+ reabsorption by intercolated cells is not completely understood.

■ REGULATION OF NaCl AND WATER REABSORPTION

Starling Forces

One of the most important factors regulating the reabsorption of solutes and water across the proximal tubule and Henle's loop are Starling forces.* These forces are illustrated in Figure 4-13. As previously described, Na^+, Cl^-, HCO_3^-, amino acids, glucose, and water are transported into the intercellular space of the proximal tubule. Starling forces between this space and the peritubular capillaries facilitate the movement of the reabsorbate into the capillaries. Starling forces that favor movement from the interstitium into the peritubular capillaries are the capillary oncotic pressure (π_{cap}) and the hydrostatic pressure in the intercellular space (P_{IS}). The opposing Starling forces are the interstitial oncotic pressure (π_{IS}) and the capillary hydrostatic pressure (P_{cap}). Normally, the sum of the Starling forces favors movement of solutes and water from the interstitium into the capillary. However, some of the solutes and fluid entering the lateral intercellular space leak back into the proximal tubular fluid (see Figure 4-13). Starling forces do not affect transport by the distal tubule and collecting duct because the water permeability of these segments is low relative to that in the proximal tubule.

Starling forces across the peritubular capillaries surrounding the proximal tubule are readily altered. Dilation of the efferent arteriole increases P_{cap}, whereas constriction of the arteriole decreases P_{cap}. An increase in P_{cap} inhibits solute and water reabsorption by increasing the back leak across the tight junction, whereas a decrease in P_{cap} stimulates reabsorption by decreasing back leak across the tight junction.

The oncotic pressure in the peritubular capillary is determined in part by the rate of formation of the glomerular ultrafiltrate (Figure 4-14). Assuming a constant plasma flow in the afferent arteriole, as less ultrafiltrate is formed (i.e., as GFR decreases), the plasma proteins become less concentrated in the plasma entering the efferent arteriole and peritubular capillary, thereby decreasing the peritubular oncotic pressure. Thus, the *peritubular oncotic pressure is directly related to the filtration fraction (FF = GFR/RPF).* A fall in the FF (in the present example due to a decrease in GFR at constant

---

*Starling forces across the walls of the peritubular capillaries are the hydrostatic pressure in the peritubular capillary (P_{cap}) and lateral intercellular space (P_{LIS}), and the oncotic pressure in the peritubular capillary (π_{cap}) and lateral intercellular space (π_{LIS}). Thus, the reabsorption of water, resulting from sodium transport from tubular fluid into the lateral intercellular space, is modified by Starling forces. Thus:

$$Q = K_f(P_{IS} - P_{cap}) - (\pi_{cap} - \pi_{IS})$$

where: Q = flow (positive numbers indicate flow from the intercellular space into blood).

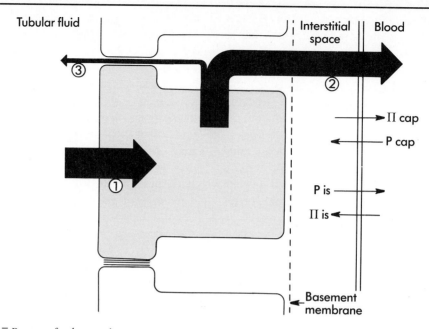

Figure 4-13 ■ Routes of solute and water transport across the proximal tubule and the Starling forces that modify reabsorption. *(1)* indicates the amount of solute and water moving across the apical membrane. This solute and water then cross the lateral cell membrane where some reenters the tubule fluid (indicate by arrow labeled *3*) and the remainder enters the interstitium and then flows into the capillary (indicated by arrow labeled *2*). Starling forces across the capillary wall determine the amount of fluid flowing through pathways *2* versus *3*. Transport mechanisms in the apical cell membranes determine the amount of solute and water entering the cell (pathway *1*). *Πcap,* capillary oncotic pressure; *Pcap,* capillary hydrostatic pressure; *Πis,* interstitial oncotic pressure; *Pis,* interstitial hydrostatic pressure. Arrows indicate direction of water movement in response to each force.

RPF) will decrease the peritubular capillary oncotic pressure. This will in turn increase back leak of solutes and water from the lateral intercellular space into the tubular fluid, thereby decreasing net solute and water reabsorption across the proximal tubule. An increase in the FF has the opposite effect.

Glomerulotubular Balance

The importance of Starling forces in regulating solute and water reabsorption by the proximal tubule is underscored by the phenomenon of *glomerulotubular balance (G-T balance).* Spontaneous changes in GFR markedly alter the filtered load of sodium (filtered load = GFR ×

P_{Na^+}). Unless such changes are rapidly accompanied by adjustments in Na^+ reabsorption, urine Na^+ excretion fluctuates widely and disturbs whole body Na^+ balance. However, spontaneous changes in GFR do not alter Na^+ balance because of G-T balance. G-T balance refers to the fact that, when body Na^+ balance is normal, Na^+ and water reabsorption increase parallel to an increase in GFR and filtered load of Na^+. Thus, a constant fraction of the filtered Na^+ and water is reabsorbed in the proximal tubule despite variations in GFR. The net result of G-T balance is a reduction of the impact of GFR changes on the amount of Na^+ and water excreted in the urine.

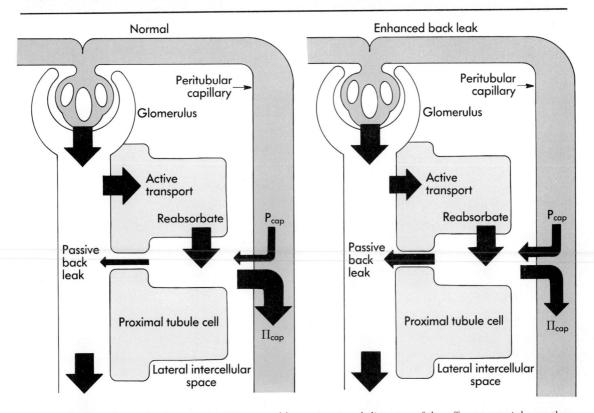

Figure 4-14 ■ Effects of a decrease in GFR, caused by an increased diameter of the efferent arteriole, on the Starling forces across the peritubular capillary and the ensuing effects on the passive back leak of solutes and water across the tight junctions of the proximal tubule. **A,** Normal. **B,** Enhanced back leak. Dilation of the efferent arteriole decrease hydrostatic pressure in the glomerular capillary, resulting in a fall in GFR. Efferent arteriole dilation also causes an increase in the hydrostatic pressure of the peritubular capillary (P_{cap}) and a fall in the oncotic pressure of the peritubular capillary (Π_{cap}). This increases the passive back leak of solutes and water across the tight junction, thereby reducing net solute and water reabsorption. Width of arrows is proportional to amount of water movement.

Two mechanisms are responsible for G-T balance: one is related to the oncotic and hydrostatic pressures between the peritubular capillaries and the lateral intercellular space (i.e., Starling forces), and the other is related to the filtered load of glucose and amino acids. As an example of the first mechanism, an increase in GFR (at constant RPF) raises the protein concentration above normal in the glomerular capillary plasma. This protein-rich plasma leaves the glomerular capillaries, flows through the efferent arteriole, and enters the peritubular capillaries.

The increased oncotic pressure in the peritubular capillaries augments the movement of solutes and fluid from the lateral intercellular space into the peritubular capillaries, thereby increasing net solute and water reabsorption.

The second mechanism responsible for G-T balance is initiated by an increase in the filtered load of glucose and amino acids. As previously discussed, the reabsorption of Na^+ is coupled with that of glucose and amino acids. The rate of Na^+ reabsorption therefore depends in part on the filtered load of glucose and amino acids.

As GFR and the filtered load of glucose and amino acids increase, Na^+ and water reabsorption also rise.

In addition to G-T balance, another physiological mechanism minimizes changes in filtered load of Na^+. As described in Chapter 3, an increase in GFR and thus in the amount of Na^+ filtered by the glomerulus activates the tubuloglomerular feedback mechanism, which returns GFR and Na^+ filtration to normal. Thus, spontaneous changes in GFR (e.g., due to changes in posture) only temporarily (minutes) increase the amount of Na^+ filtered. Until GFR returns to normal, the mechanisms that underlie G-T balance keep urinary sodium excretion constant and thereby maintain Na^+ homeostasis (see Chapter 6).

Hormones

Table 4-5 summarizes the effects of several hormones on Na^+, Cl^-, and water reabsorption by the nephron segments. All of the hormones listed in this table act within minutes, except aldosterone, which delays its action on Na^+ reabsorption for 1 hour. The regulation by these hormones of K^+, Ca^{++}, PO_4^{3-}, and Mg^{++} reabsorption are described in Chapters 7 and 9.

Sympathetic Nervous System

The sympathetic nervous system also regulates Na^+, Cl^-, and water reabsorption by the proximal tubule and Henle's loop. Activation of sympathetic nerves (e.g., after volume depletion) stimulates reabsorption, whereas inhibition of these nerves has the opposite effect.

■ KEY WORDS AND CONCEPTS

- Reabsorption
- Secretion
- Passive diffusion
- Facilitated diffusion
- Uniport, symport, and antiport
- Secondary active transport

Table 4-5 ■ Hormones that regulate NaCl and water reabsorption

Segment	Hormone	Effects on NaCl and water reabsorption	
Proximal Tubule			
	Angiotensin II	↑ NaCl	↑ H_2O
	Glucocorticoids	↑ NaCl	↑ H_2O
Thick Ascending Limb			
	Aldosterone	↑ NaCl	
	Vasopressin	↑ NaCl	
Distal Tubule/Collecting Duct			
	Aldosterone	↑ NaCl	
	Atrial natriuretic peptide	↓ NaCl	↓ H_2O
	Prostaglandins	↓ NaCl	↓ H_2O
	Bradykinin	↓ NaCl	
	Vasopressin	↑ NaCl	↑ H_2O

- Active transport
- Endocytosis
- Solvent drag
- Coupled transport
- Tight junction
- Lateral intercellular space
- Transcellular pathway
- Paracellular pathway
- Water reabsorption is secondary to solute transport
- Glomerulotubular balance
- Starling forces

■ SELF-STUDY PROBLEMS

1. Consider the amount of water and NaCl filtered and reabsorbed by the kidneys each day. What does this tell you about the amount of energy (ATP) expended by the kidneys? Could this explain why the blood flow is so high relative to the size of the kidneys?

2. What is the composition and volume of a normal 24-hour urine?

3. Compare and contrast passive and active transport.

4. If it were possible to completely inhibit Na^+-K^+-ATPase in the kidney, what would happen to transcellular and paracellular NaCl reabsorption across the proximal tubule? If GFR was unchanged, how much water and NaCl would appear in the urine each day?

5. Describe the mechanisms and pathways of Na^+, glucose, amino acid, Cl^-, and water reabsorption by the proximal tubule. Which pathways occur in the first phase of reabsorption, and which occur in the second? How do Starling forces affect solute and water reabsorption?

6. Describe how Na^+ and Cl^- are reabsorbed by the thick ascending limb of Henle's loop. If a diuretic that inhibits NaCl reabsorption (e.g., furosemide) in the thick ascending limb was given to an individual, what would happen to water reabsorption by this segment?

7. What is glomerulotubular balance, and what is the physiological significance of this phenomenon? What would happen to Na^+ balance if glomerulotubular balance did not exist?

8. List the hormones and factors that regulate NaCl and water reabsorption by each segment of the nephron.

5 Regulation of Body Fluid Osmolality

■ OBJECTIVES

1. Explain the osmotic and hemodynamic control of antidiuretic hormone (ADH) secretion.
2. Describe the cellular events associated with the action of ADH on the collecting duct cells, and how they lead to an increase in the water permeability of this segment.
3. Explain the process of countercurrent multiplication by Henle's loop, and how it allows the single effect of separating solute and water to dilute and concentrate the urine.
4. Explain the importance of the medullary interstitium in the production of a concentrated urine, and the role of the vasa recta in maintaining the medullary interstitial osmotic gradient for NaCl and urea.
5. Quantitate the diluting and concentrating ability of the kidneys in terms of solute-free water.

The body loses water by several routes, including the lungs during respiration; the skin by perspiration; the gastrointestinal tract in the feces; and the kidneys in the urine.* The kidneys are the most important route, because renal water excretion is regulated to keep the osmolality of the body fluids constant.

It is important to recognize that water balance disorders are manifested by alterations in body fluid osmolality (e.g., plasma). Because the major determinant of plasma osmolality is Na^+ (with its anions Cl^- and HCO_3^-), these disor-

ders result in alterations in the plasma $[Na^+]$. When evaluating an abnormal plasma $[Na^+]$ in an individual, it is tempting to suspect a problem in Na^+ balance. However, the problem relates to water balance, not Na^+ balance. As described in Chapter 6, changes in Na^+ balance result in alterations in the volume of extracellular fluid, not its osmolality.

When water intake is low, or when it is lost from the body by other routes (e.g., perspiration, diarrhea), the kidneys conserve water by producing a small volume of urine that is hyperosmotic with respect to plasma. When water intake is high, a large volume of hyposmotic urine is produced. In a normal individual, urine osmolality can vary from approximately 50 to 1,200 mOsm/kg H_2O, and urine volume can

---

*The loss of water via the lungs, skin, and gastrointestinal tract is collectively termed "insensible water loss" because of the difficulty associated with its measurement. In a normal individual, insensible water loss is approximately 1 to 1.2 L/day.

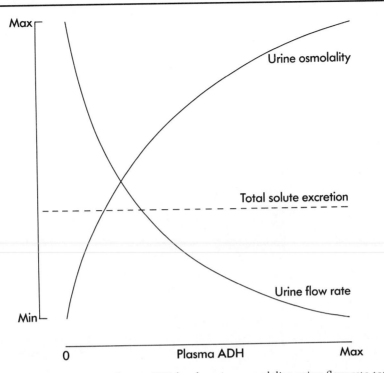

Figure 5-1 ■ Relationship between plasma ADH levels, urine osmolality, urine flow rate total solute excretion.

vary from as much as 20 L/day to as little as 0.5 L/day.

The kidneys are capable of controlling water excretion independently of their ability to control the excretion of a number of other physiologically significant substances (e.g., Na$^+$, K$^+$, H$^+$, and urea). Indeed this ability is necessary for survival, because it allows water balance to be achieved without upsetting the other homeostatic functions of the kidneys.

This chapter discusses the mechanisms by which the kidneys excrete either hyposmotic (dilute) or hyperosmotic (concentrated) urine. The control of vasopressin secretion and its important role in regulating the excretion of water by the kidneys is also explained.

■ ANTIDIURETIC HORMONE

Antidiuretic hormone (ADH), or vasopressin, acts on the kidneys to regulate the volume and

osmolality of the urine. When plasma ADH levels are low, a large volume of urine is excreted *(diuresis)*, and the urine is dilute. When plasma levels are high, a small volume of urine is excreted *(antidiuresis)*, and the urine is concentrated.* Figure 5-1 illustrates the effect of ADH on the urine flow rate and the osmolality of this urine. The excretion of total solute (e.g., Na$^+$, K$^+$, H$^+$, and urea) by the kidneys is also shown. Note that ADH does not appreciably alter the excretion of solute. This underscores the fact that ADH controls water excretion and maintains water balance without altering the excretion and homeostatic control of other substances.

---

*Diuresis is simply a large urine output. When urine contains primarily water, it is referred to as water diuresis. This is in contrast to the diuresis seen with diuretic agents (see Chapter 10). In the latter case, there is a large urine output, but the urine contains solute and water.

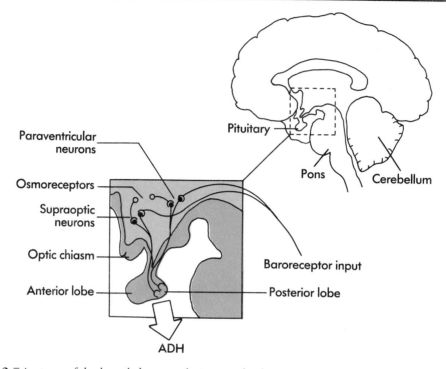

Figure 5-2 ■ Anatomy of the hypothalamus and pituitary gland. Depicted is the relationship between the ADH neurosecretory cells, the osmoreceptors, and input from the vascular baroreceptors.

ADH is a small peptide that is 9 amino acids in length. It is synthesized in neuroendocrine cells located within the *supraoptic* and *paraventricular nuclei* of the hypothalamus. The synthesized hormone is packaged in granules that are transported down the axon of the cell and stored in the nerve terminals located in the *neurohypophysis (posterior pituitary)*. The anatomy of the hypothalamus and pituitary gland are shown in Figure 5-2.

The secretion of ADH by the posterior pituitary can be influenced by several factors. The two primary physiological regulators of ADH secretion are osmotic (plasma osmolality) and hemodynamic (blood volume and pressure). Other factors that can alter ADH secretion are nausea (stimulates), atrial natriuretic hormone (inhibits), and angiotensin II (stimulates). A number of drugs, prescription and nonprescrip-

tion, also affect ADH secretion. For example, nicotine stimulates secretion, whereas ethanol inhibits it.

Osmotic Control of ADH Secretion

Changes in the osmolality of body fluids play the most important role in regulating ADH secretion; changes as minor as 1% are sufficient to significantly alter it. Cells located in the hypothalamus, excluding those that synthesize ADH, sense changes in body fluid osmolality. These cells, termed *osmoreceptors*, appear to behave as osmometers and sense changes in osmolality by either shrinking or swelling. It is important to recognize that the osmoreceptors respond only to solutes in plasma that are *effective osmoles* (see Chapter 1). For example, urea is an *ineffective osmole* when considering the function of the osmoreceptors. Thus, ele-

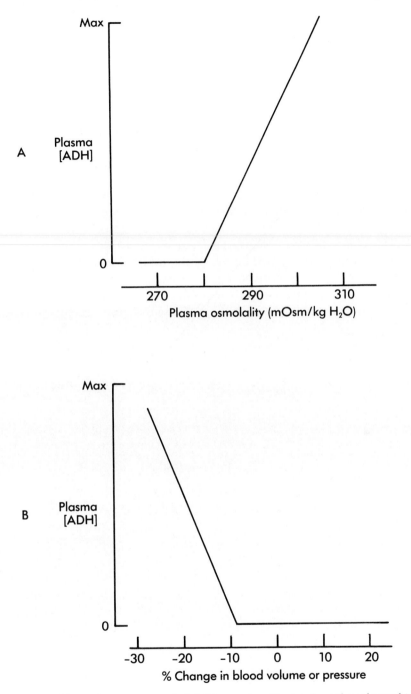

Figure 5-3 ■ Osmotic and hemodynamic control of ADH secretion. Depicted are the relationships between plasma ADH levels, and plasma osmolality *(A)*, and blood volume and pressure *(B)*.

vation of the plasma urea concentration alone will have little effect on ADH secretion.

When the effective osmolality of plasma increases, the osmoreceptors send signals to the ADH synthesizing cells located in the supraoptic and paraventricular nuclei of the hypothalamus, and ADH secretion is stimulated. Conversely, when the effective osmolality of plasma is reduced, secretion is inhibited. Because ADH is rapidly degraded in plasma, circulating levels can be reduced to zero within minutes after secretion is inhibited. As a result, the ADH system can respond rapidly to fluctuations in plasma osmolality.

Figure 5-3, *A* illustrates the effect of changes in plasma osmolality on circulating ADH levels. The slope of the relationship is quite steep and accounts for the sensitivity of this system. The *set point* of the system is the plasma osmolality

value at which ADH secretion begins to increase. Below this set point, virtually no ADH is released. The set point varies between individuals and is genetically determined. In healthy adults, it varies from 280 to 290 mOsm/kg H_2O. Several physiological factors can change the set point in a given individual. As discussed below, alterations in blood volume and pressure can shift it. In addition, pregnancy is associated with a decrease in the set point.

Hemodynamic Control of ADH Secretion

A decrease in blood volume or pressure also stimulates ADH secretion. The receptors responsible for this reponse are located in both the low-pressure (left atrium and pulmonary vessels) and high-pressure (aortic arch and carotid sinus) sides of the circulatory system. These receptors, called *baroreceptors*, respond

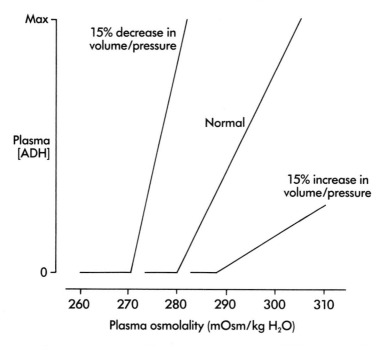

Figure 5-4 ■ Interaction between osmotic and hemodynamic stimuli for ADH secretion. With decreased blood volume and pressure, the osmotic set point is shifted to lower plasma osmolality values and the slope is increased. An increase in blood volume and pressure has the opposite effects.

to stretch (see Chapter 6). Signals from baro-receptors are relayed to the ADH secretory cells of the supraoptic and paraventricular hypotha-lamic nuclei via afferent fibers in the vagus and glossopharyngeal nerves. The sensitivity of the baroreceptor system is less than that of the os-moreceptors, and a 5% to 10% decrease in blood volume or pressure is required before ADH secretion is stimulated. This is illustrated in Figure 5-3, *B*.

Alterations in blood volume and pressure also affect the response to changes in body fluid os-molality (Figure 5-4). With a decrease in blood volume or pressure, the set point is shifted to lower osmolality values, and the slope of the relationship is steeper. In terms of survival of the individual, this means that, faced with cir-culatory collapse, the kidneys will continue to conserve water, even though they reduce the osmolality of body fluids. With an increase in blood volume or pressure, the opposite occurs.

The set point is shifted to higher osmolality val-ues, and the slope is decreased.

ADH Actions on the Kidneys

ADH exerts two primary actions on the kid-neys: It stimulates NaCl reabsorption by the thick ascending limb of Henle's loop and in-creases the permeability of the collecting duct to water and urea. (The effect on urea is limited to the portion of the collecting duct located in the inner medulla.)

The cellular events associated with ADH-stimulated transport by the thick ascending limb have not been completely explained. However, it is known that net reabsorption of NaCl is in-creased as a result of stimulated activity of the $1Na^+, 2Cl^-, 1K^+$ symporter located in the apical membrane of the cell. This augments the ability of the kidneys to concentrate the urine.

The actions of ADH on the water permeability of the collecting duct have been extensively

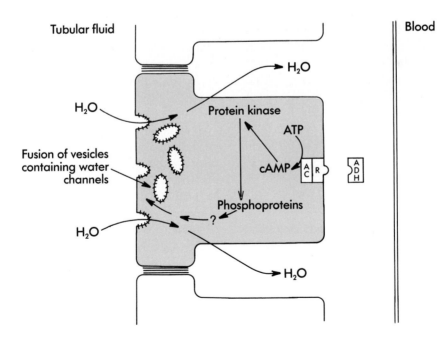

Figure 5-5 ■ Cellular events associated with action of ADH on the principal cells of the collecting duct. *R*, ADH receptor; *AC*, adenylyl cyclase. See text for details.

studied. Figure 5-5 is a simplified scheme of current knowledge in this regard. ADH binds to a receptor on the basolateral membrane of the cell. Binding to this receptor, which is coupled to *adenylyl cyclase*, increases the intracellular levels of *cyclic adenosine monophosphate (cAMP)*. The rise in intracellular cAMP activates one or more *protein kinases*, which results in the insertion of vesicles containing *water channels* into the apical membrane of the cell. These water channels are preformed and reside in vesicles located beneath the cell's apical membrane. With the removal of ADH, these water channels are reinternalized into the cell, and the apical membrane is once again impermeable to water. This shuttling of water channels into and out of the apical membrane provides a rapid mechanism for controlling membrane water permeability. Because the basolateral membrane is freely permeable to water, any water that enters the cell through the apical membrane water channels will exit across the basolateral membrane, resulting in the net absorption of water from the tubule lumen.

ADH also increases the urea permeability of the inner medullary portion of the collecting duct. When ADH binds to its membrane receptor, cAMP levels within the inner medullary collecting duct cells rise. Ultimately, and by mechanisms not yet defined, this rise in intracellular cAMP activates specific urea transporters in the membrane, and thereby urea permeability is increased.

Disorders of ADH Secretion and Action

In the absence of ADH, the kidneys are unable to concentrate the urine, and the individual excretes large volumes of dilute urine *(polyuria)*. With complete absence of ADH, it is not uncommon for urine output to exceed 10 L/day. To compensate for this loss of water, the individual must drink comparable volumes of water *(polydipsia)*. Individuals who lack ADH, or whose kidneys do not respond to this hor-

mone, are said to have *diabetes insipidus*. This disorder can result from inadequate ADH secretion by the posterior pituitary *(central diabetes insipidus)*, or a failure of the collecting duct to respond to ADH *(nephrogenic diabetes insipidus)*.

Central diabetes insipidus is a rare genetic abnormality, but it is seen more commonly after head trauma, with brain neoplasms, or with brain infections. Nephrogenic diabetes insipidus is associated with some metabolic disorders (e.g., hypercalcemia), or with administration of some drugs (e.g., Li^+). Individuals with diabetes insipidus can develop life-threatening hyperosmolality if their access to water is restricted.

ADH can be elevated above levels expected from either the plasma osmolality or the blood volume and pressure. This condition of non-physiological release of ADH is termed *syndrome of inappropriate secretion of ADH (SIADH)*. It is a common clinical problem with multiple causes, including brain infections and neoplasms, pulmonary infections and neoplasms, and a large number of drugs (e.g., antitumor drugs). Individuals with SIADH have reduced plasma osmolality and inappropriately concentrated urine.

■ THIRST

In addition to affecting the secretion of ADH, changes in plasma osmolality and blood volume or pressure lead to alterations in the perception of thirst. When body fluid osmolality is increased or the blood volume or pressure is reduced, the individual perceives thirst. Of these stimuli, hypertonicity is the most potent. An increase in plasma osmolality of only 2% to 3% will produce a strong desire to drink, while decreases in blood volume and pressure in the range of 10% to 15% are required to provoke the same response.

The neural centers involved with the thirst response have not been completely defined. It appears that osmoreceptors similar to, but distinct from, those involved in vasopressin release respond to changes in plasma osmolality. Like the vasopressin osmoreceptors, those involved in thirst respond only to effective osmoles. Even less is known about the pathways involved in the thirst response to decreased blood volume or pressure, but it is believed that they may be the same as those involved in the vasopressin system.

The sensation of thirst is satisfied by the act of drinking even before sufficient water is absorbed from the gastrointestinal tract to correct the plasma osmolality. Oropharyngeal and upper gastrointestinal receptors appear to be involved in this response. However, relief of the thirst sensation via these receptors is short-lived, and thirst is only completely satisfied when plasma osmolality or blood volume or pressure is corrected.

It should be apparent that *the ADH and thirst systems work in concert to maintain water balance*. An increase in plasma osmolality invokes drinking and, via ADH action on the kidneys, the conservation of water. Conversely, when plasma osmolality is decreased, thirst is suppressed and, in the absence of ADH, renal water excretion is enhanced.

■ COUNTERCURRENT MULTIPLICATION BY HENLE'S LOOP

The production of urine that is hyposmotic or hyperosmotic with respect to plasma requires solute to be separated from water at some point along the nephron. The production of hyposmotic urine is conceptually easy to understand. The nephron must simply reabsorb solute from the tubular fluid and not allow water to follow. As will be explained, this can occur under appropriate conditions in the ascending limb of Henle's loop, the distal tubule, and the collecting duct.

The excretion of a hyperosmotic urine is more complicated. This process requires the removal of water from the tubular fluid, leaving solute behind. Because water can only move passively, driven by an osmotic gradient, the kidneys must be able to generate a hyperosmotic environment that can be used to remove water from the tubular fluid. Indeed, such an environment is generated in the renal medulla. Henle's loop is critical for generating this hyperosmotic medullary environment. The importance of Henle's loop in the production of hyperosmotic urine is underscored by the fact that, while the kidneys of all vertebrates can produce dilute urine, only the kidneys of birds and mammals, can develop hyperosmotic urine, and only their kidneys possess Henle's loops. The key to understanding how Henle's loop functions in this regard is recognizing its ability to operate as a *countercurrent multiplier* (see Figure 5-6).

Henle's loop consists of two parallel limbs with tubular fluid flowing in opposite directions *(countercurrent flow)*. Fluid flows into the medulla in the descending limb and out of the medulla in the ascending limb. In the idealized situation portrayed in Figure 5-6, fluid within both limbs and the surrounding interstitial fluid have an initial osmolality equal to that of plasma (300 mOsm/kg H_2O).* The ascending limb is impermeable to water and reabsorbs solute from the luminal fluid. Thus, fluid within this limb becomes diluted. This separation of solute and water by the ascending limb is termed the *single effect* of the countercurrent multiplication process. The solute removed from the ascending limb tubular fluid accumulates in the surrounding interstitial fluid and raises its osmolality.

The descending limb has very different permeability characteristics. Specifically, it has a high water permeability and a low solute permeability. Consequently, the hyperosmotic medullary interstitium causes water to move

---

*Plasma osmolality is normally near 290 mOsm/kg H_2O; however, we will assume a value of 300 mOsm/kg H_2O for simplicity.

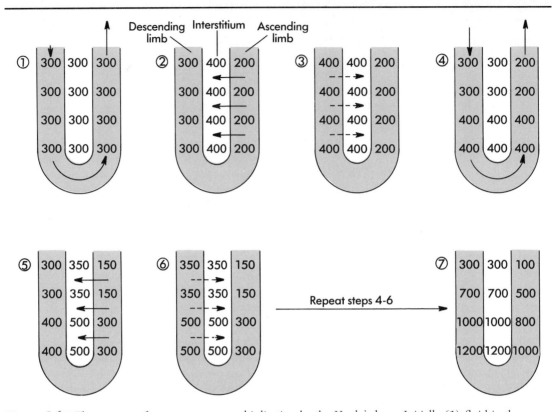

Figure 5-6 ■ The process of countercurrent multiplication by the Henle's loop. Initially *(1)*, fluid in the Henle's loop and interstitium has an osmolality equal to plasma (300 mOsm/kg H$_2$O). The transport of solute out of the ascending limb into the interstitium represents the single effect of separating solute from water *(2 and 5)*. The osmotic pressure gradient between the interstitium and the descending limb results in passive movement of water out of the descending limb *(3 and 6)*. In the steady state, with continuous tubular fluid flow *(4)*, the single effect is multiplied along the length of the loop establishing a standing osmotic gradient *(7)*.

out of the descending limb. With equilibration, the osmolality of the tubular fluid within the descending limb will equal that of the surrounding interstitial fluid. As depicted in Figure 5-6, the net effect of this process is the establishment of a 200 mOsm/kg H$_2$O osmotic gradient between the tubular fluid in the ascending and descending limbs.

Henle's loop is not a static system, since fresh tubular fluid constantly enters the descending limb from the proximal tubule. Because proximal tubular reabsorption is an isosmotic process

(see Chapter 4), the osmolality of this entering fluid is equal to that of plasma. As this fluid flows into the descending limb, the hyperosmotic fluid in the descending limb flows into the ascending limb. Separation of solute from water again occurs in the ascending limb, which leads to the reestablishment of the 200 mOsm/kg H$_2$O osmotic gradient between the two limbs. With sufficient time, and in the steady state, the situation depicted in Panel 7 of Figure 5-6 results. Ultimately, the single effect of separating solute from water is multiplied by the countercurrent flow of fluid in the loop, such that the fluid at the bend of the loop is hyperosmotic to plasma. Also, a standing interstitial fluid osmotic gradient is established from the junction of the medulla and cortex to the papilla.

As illustrated in Panel 7 of Figure 5-6, fluid with an osmolality of 300 mOsm/kg H_2O enters the medulla in the descending limb of Henle's loop, and fluid with an osmolality of 100 mOsm/kg H_2O exits the loop in the ascending limb. For mass balance to exist, there must be another route for solute to leave the medulla. As will be further described, this occurs by way of the collecting duct (hyperosmotic urine) and the ascending vasa recta.

Clearly, countercurrent multiplication is an energy-efficient process whereby a considerable osmotic gradient is generated between fluid in the tip of Henle's loop and systemic plasma ($1,200 - 300 = 900$ mOsm/kg H_2O). The cost in energy of establishing this gradient is modest and only represents the energy expended in generating the 200 mOsm/kg H_2O gradient between adjacent segments of the descending and ascending limbs.

To understand how the process of countercurrent multiplication results in the excretion of dilute or concentrated urine, it is necessary to consider in some detail the following:

1. The transport and permeability properties of the various portions of Henle's loop, the distal tubule, and collecting duct.
2. The importance of the medullary interstitial osmotic gradient.
3. The function of the vasa recta.
4. The transition from a diuretic to an antidiuretic state, and the vital role of ADH.

Transport and Permeability Properties of the Nephron Segments

As discussed in Chapter 4, the proximal tubule reabsorbs solute and water by a process that is essentially isosmotic, regardless of whether dilute or concentrated urine is produced. Thus, no separation of solute and water takes place in the proximal tubule. Consequently, to understand the processes involved in the dilution and concentration of urine, focus must be turned to all nephron segments distal to the proximal tubule (Figure 5-7).

As noted, dilute urine is produced when plasma ADH levels are low. Figure 5-7, *D* shows that, under this condition (solid lines), all tubule segments except the descending thin limb of Henle's loop have a very low water permeability. Reabsorption of solute (NaCl) by these segments (Figure 5-7, *A*) therefore dilutes the luminal fluid. Because of its large transport capacity, the thick ascending limb of Henle's loop is the major site of tubular fluid dilution. Indeed, the thick ascending limb of Henle's loop is often referred to as the *diluting segment* of the kidney.

Figure 5-7 points out some other important features of these nephron segments. First, with the exception of the ascending thin limb of Henle's loop and outer medullary portion of the descending limb of Henle's loop, the passive NaCl permeability of these nephron segments is quite low (see Fig. 5-7, *B*). The relatively high NaCl permeability of the ascending thin limb, coupled with the high [NaCl] in the tubular fluid (see below), allows for passive efflux of NaCl out of the tubule lumen. Because this segment is also impermeable to water, the efflux of NaCl results in separation of solute and water, and thus dilution of the luminal fluid. Second, only the nephron segments deep within the medulla have significant passive urea permeabilities (Figure 5-7, *C*). This allows urea to be accumulated in the inner medulla, which is a critical requirement for maximal urine concentrating ability.

Medullary Interstitial Osmotic Gradient

The medullary interstitium plays a critical role in the urine concentrating and diluting process. The osmolality of this fluid provides the driving force for the absorption of water from

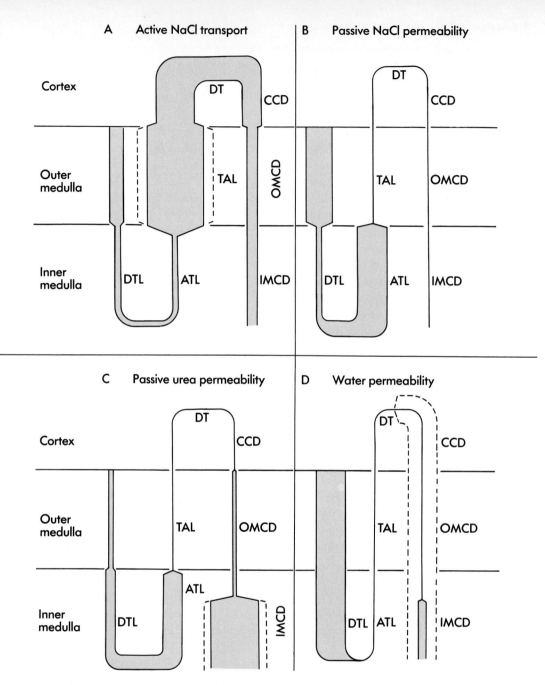

Figure 5-7 ■ Transport and passive permeability properties of the nephron segments involved in the dilution and concentration of the urine. The width of the tubular segments is proportional to the magnitude of the parameter. The solid lines depict the situation in the absence of ADH. The dashed lines shows the effect of ADH. DTL, descending thin limb; ATL, ascending thin limb; *TAL*, thick ascending limb; *DT*, distal tubule; *CCD*, cortical collecting duct; *OMCD*, outer medullary collecting duct; *IMCD*, inner medullary collecting duct. (Adapted from Knepper MA and Rector FC Jr: Urinary concentration and dilution. In Brenner BM and Rector FC Jr (editors): The kidney, ed 4, Philadelphia, 1991, WB Saunders Co.)

the descending thin limb of Henle's loop and the terminal portions of the collecting duct.

Measurements of the composition of the medullary interstitial fluid have shown that its principal constituents are NaCl and urea, and that the distribution of these solutes is not uniform throughout the medulla.* At the junction of the cortex and outer medulla, the interstitial fluid has an osmolality similar to that of plasma (300 mOsm/kg H_2O), with nearly all osmoles attributable to NaCl. Interstitial fluid osmolality rises progressively with increasing depth into the medulla and attains a value of approximately 1,200 mOsm/kg H_2O at the papilla. At this point, the distribution of osmoles is roughly 600 mOsm/kg H_2O due to NaCl, and 600 mOsm/kg H_2O due to urea.

This *medullary interstitial osmotic gradient* for NaCl and urea is generated by the processes of countercurrent multiplication and urea trapping. In the previous section, the role of countercurrent multiplication in producing the medullary interstitial osmotic gradient was explained. This process applies to the accumulation of NaCl, which is deposited in the interstitium as a result of transport out of the lumen of the thin and thick ascending limbs of Henle's loop. The process of medullary urea accumulation is more complex, however, and requires consideration of the urea permeability properties of the various nephron segments (see Figure 5-7, *C*).

Urea enters the tubule by glomerular filtration. A portion of this filtered load of urea is reabsorbed into the blood by the proximal tubule. However, this occurs with water, such that the [urea] in the tubular fluid entering the me-

dulla in the descending limb of Henle's loop is nearly equal to that in plasma. As indicated in Figure 5-7, *C*, of the remaining nephron segments, only the inner medullary collecting duct has a high urea permeability. (The lower, but significant permeabilities of the descending thin and ascending thin limbs of Henle's loop will be discussed below.) Consequently, most of the urea that enters the descending thin limb of Henle's loop from the proximal tubule remains trapped in the tubule lumen until it reaches the inner medullary collecting duct. At this point, some urea can leave the lumen of the inner medullary collecting duct and enter the medullary interstitium. Note that the movement of urea is passive and occurs in the direction of a favorable urea concentration gradient.

In the presence of ADH, water reabsorption from the tubular fluid across the cortical and outer medullary portions of the collecting duct causes the [urea] in tubular fluid to rise. When this fluid reaches the inner medullary collecting duct, urea diffuses out of the tubule into the interstitium. In the absence of ADH, fluid reaching the inner medullary collecting duct is dilute and has a low [urea]. As a result, under this condition, urea will diffuse from the medullary interstitium into the lumen of the collecting duct. However, this diffusion (i.e., urea secretion) is limited by the reduced urea permeability of the inner medullary collecting duct in the absence of ADH.

Both the descending thin and ascending thin limbs of Henle's loop are permeable to urea, although permeability is less than that of the inner medullary collecting duct (see Figure 5-7, *C*). Normally, the [urea] in both of these segments is less than that in the surrounding interstitial fluid. Consequently, urea enters the tubular fluid at these sites. This recycling of urea (exit from the inner medullary collecting duct and entry into the thin limbs of Henle's loop) aids in the trapping and accumulation of urea in the inner medullary interstitium.

---

*As noted in Chapter 1, urea can be an ineffective osmole. This is the case for cells that have a high urea permeability due to the presence of a specific urea transporter in their plasma membranes (e.g., red blood cells). However, urea does behave as an effective osmole in most of the segments of the distal nephron; Therefore, in these segments, urea causes osmotic water flow.

As previously described, the hyperosmotic medullary interstitium is vital to the process of countercurrent multiplication, specifically the reabsorption of water from the descending thin limb of Henle's loop. The hyperosmotic medullary interstitium is also essential for concentrating the tubular fluid within the collecting duct. Due to the hyperosmotic medullary interstitium and in the presence of ADH, water is reabsorbed from the collecting duct, driven by the osmotic gradient between the luminal fluid and the interstitium. Because water movement out of the collecting duct is passive, the osmolality of the medullary interstitium defines the maximum urine osmolality. For example, if the osmolality of the interstitial fluid at the papilla is 1,200 mOsm/kg H_2O, the osmolality of the urine can equal but not exceed this value. (Note

that urine osmolality can be less than that of the interstitium; this will occur with less than maximal ADH levels.)

Because a hyperosmotic medullary interstitium is essential for concentrating urine, any process that reduces this osmolality will result in the inability to maximally concentrate urine. For example, if the medullary interstitium osmolality were reduced to 800 mOsm/kg H_2O, the maximum osmolality of the urine would also be 800 mOsm/kg H_2O.

Vasa Recta Function: Countercurrent Exchange

As described in Chapter 2, the blood supply to the renal medulla consists of *vasa recta*, which run parallel to Henle's loop. The vasa recta serve two important functions: They pro-

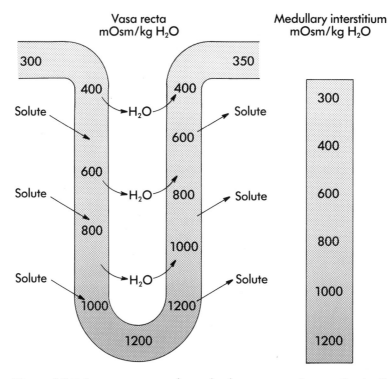

Figure 5-8 ■ Countercurrent exchange by the vasa recta. See text for details.

vide nutrients and oxygen to the tubules in the medulla, and, more importantly, help maintain the medullary interstitial osmotic gradient by acting as *countercurrent exchangers*. As countercurrent exchangers, the vasa recta remove the excess water and solute added to the medullary interstitium by the various nephron segments in the medulla, which would otherwise dissipate the gradient. This process is illustrated in Figure 5-8.

Plama entering the medulla via the descending vasa recta has an osmolality equal to that of the systemic plasma (300 mOsm/kg H_2O). As it flows deeper into the medulla, it achieves balance with the surrounding interstitial fluid by gaining solute and losing water (the vasa recta have high permeabilities to both solute and water). At the papilla, it will have an osmolality equal to that of the surrounding interstitium (e.g., 1,200 mOsm/kg H_2O). If the vasa recta were to exit the medulla at this point, they would reduce the osmolality of the interstitium by removing the accumulated solutes. However, because of countercurrent flow, the blood reequilibrates as it ascends back through the medulla. As a result, the plasma exiting the medulla in the ascending vasa recta is only slightly hyperosmotic compared to plasma, and the hyperosmotic medullary interstitium is preserved. The vasa recta remove the excess water and solutes that are added to the interstitial fluid by the various nephron segments in the medulla.

Diuresis vs. Antidiuresis and the Role of ADH

During the diuretic state, ADH is absent, and the nephron segments beginning with the ascending thin limb of Henle's loop and continuing on through the collecting duct have a low water permeability (see Figure 5-7, *D*). Consequently, the separation of solute from water by these nephron segments results in a dilute urine. The only change necessary for a transition to the antidiuretic state is for ADH to be present and effective. As described, the primary actions of ADH on the kidneys are to increase the water and urea permeability of the collecting duct and stimulate NaCl transport by the thick ascending limb of Henle's loop.

With regard to water permeability, ADH exerts its effect beginning at the terminal one third of the distal tubule and continuing throughout the entire collecting duct. Because the thin and thick ascending limbs of Henle's loop are impermeable to water, fluid entering the distal tubule is always hyposmotic to plasma (approximately 100 mOsm/kg H_2O), regardless of the presence of ADH. Therefore, when ADH is present, water exits the tubule lumen by osmosis into the surrounding interstitial tissue because of the existing osmotic gradient. With maximal levels of ADH, the tubular fluid comes to osmotic equilibrium with the interstitial fluid as it flows down the collecting duct. Thus, the tubular fluid in the cortex will be in osmotic equilibrium with plasma (300 mOsm/kg H_2O). At the papilla, it will have an osmolality equal to that of the surrounding medullary interstitial fluid (1,200 mOsm/kg H_2O). Because individual collecting ducts join together as they descend through the medulla, there are many more cortical collecting ducts than medullary collecting ducts. Consequently, more water is reabsorbed in the cortex than in the medulla.

ADH also acts on the thick ascending limb of Henle's loop to enhance NaCl reabsorption, and on the inner medullary collecting duct to increase urea permeability. These actions result in the accumulation of additional amounts of these solutes in the medullary interstitium. This maintains the osmotic gradient between interstitium and collecting duct lumen at a time when water reabsorption would dissipate the medullary interstitial osmotic gradient.

■ INTEGRATED VIEW OF THE URINE CONCENTRATING PROCESS

Figure 5-9 capsulizes the essential features of the urine concentrating process. As depicted, ADH levels are maximal, and a concentrated

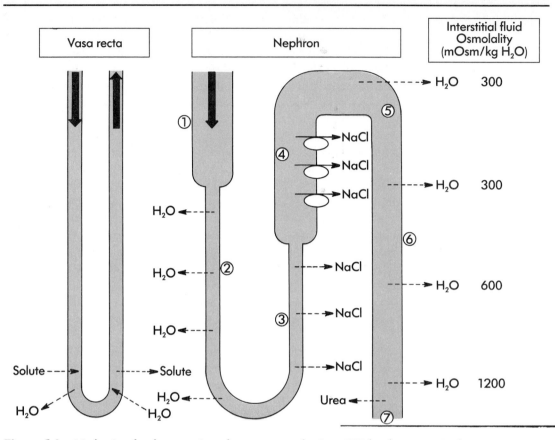

Figure 5-9 ■ Mechanism for the excretion of a concentrated urine. ADH levels are maximal. Passive movements of water and solutes are indicated by dashed lines. Numbers refer to description of process in text. NaCl is actively absorbed in the thick ascending limb of Henle's loop.

urine is excreted. The mechanisms for production of a dilute urine are the same, except ADH is not present, and therefore water is not reabsorbed from the lumen of the collecting duct.

The following steps describe the urine concentrating process (numbers correspond to those in Figure 5-9):

1. Fluid entering the descending thin limb of Henle's loop from the proximal tubule is isosmotic with respect to plasma. This reflects the isosmotic nature of solute and fluid reabsorption in the proximal tubule (see Chapter 4). The osmolality of this solution is approximately 300 mOsm/kg H_2O, with the majority of the osmoles due to NaCl.

2. The descending thin limb is highly permeable to water and much less so to NaCl and urea. Consequently, water is reabsorbed as the fluid flows deeper into the hyperosmotic medulla. By this process, fluid at the bend of the loop has an osmolality equal to that of the surrounding interstitial fluid (1,200 mOsm/kg H_2O). Most of the osmoles are due to NaCl, although the other components of the tubular fluid are concentrated as well. The [urea] of the tubular fluid also begins to increase. This is due to the reabsorption of water from the tubular fluid and the diffusion of urea into the descending

thin limb from the medullary interstitium (urea recycling).

3. The ascending thin limb is essentially impermeable to water, but permeable to NaCl. As the NaCl-rich tubular fluid moves up the ascending thin limb, NaCl passively diffuses into the medullary interstitium. (Recall that NaCl accounts for 600 mOsm/kg H_2O of the interstitial fluid osmolality, while nearly 1,000 mOsm/kg H_2O is attributable to NaCl in the tubular fluid entering the ascending thin limb.) This passive reabsorption of NaCl, without concomitant water reabsorption, will begin to dilute the tubular fluid. Because the ascending thin limb is urea permeable, urea will also diffuse from the medullary interstitium into the tubule lumen.

4. The thick ascending limb of Henle's loop is also essentially impermeable to water. Active reabsorption of NaCl by this nephron segment further dilutes the tubular fluid. As noted, ADH also stimulates the active reabsorption of NaCl by the thick ascending limb of Henle's loop. Dilution occurs to such a degree that fluid leaving this limb is hyposmotic with respect to plasma (approximately 100 mOsm/kg H_2O).

5. Fluid reaching the collecting duct is hyposmotic with respect to the surrounding interstitial fluid. Therefore, water diffuses out of the tubule lumen in the presence of ADH; this begins the process of urine concentration. The maximum osmolality attainable by the fluid in the cortical collecting duct is approximately 300 mOsm/kg H_2O, which is the osmolality of the surrounding interstitial fluid and plasma. Although at this point the fluid is the same osmolality as that which entered the descending thin limb, its composition has been dramatically altered. Because of reabsorption by the preceding nephron segments, NaCl accounts for a much smaller portion of the total tubular fluid osmolality. Instead, the tubular fluid osmolality reflects the presence of urea (filtered urea plus urea added in the descending thin and ascending thin limbs of Henle's loop) and other nonreabsorbed solutes (e.g., creatinine).

6. As fluid in the collecting duct continues through the medulla, water is reabsorbed. This increases the osmolality of the tubular fluid, which at this point is due mainly to urea. In the inner medulla, the collecting duct is permeable to urea, and ADH increases this permeability. Because the urea concentration of the tubular fluid has been increased by water reabsorption, some urea diffuses out of the tubule lumen into the medullary interstitium.

7. The urine will have an osmolality of 1,200 mOsm/kg H_2O and contain high concentrations of urea and other nonreabsorbed solutes. Because luminal fluid [urea] tends to equilibrate with the interstitial urea, its concentration in the urine will not exceed that of the interstitium (approximately 600 mmol/L). The high NaCl concentration of the interstitium drives additional water reabsorption, concentrating the other nonreabsorbed solutes in the tubular fluid.

■ QUANTITATING RENAL DILUTING AND CONCENTRATING ABILITY

The central process in the dilution and concentration of urine is the single effect of separating solute from water. Through this separation, the kidneys, in a sense, generate a volume of water that is free of all solute. When the urine is dilute, this *solute-free water* is excreted from the body. When the urine is concentrated, this water is returned to systemic circulation. The concept of *free-water clearance* provides a means for measuring the ability of the kidneys to generate solute-free water. This concept directly follows renal clearance as described in Chapter 3.

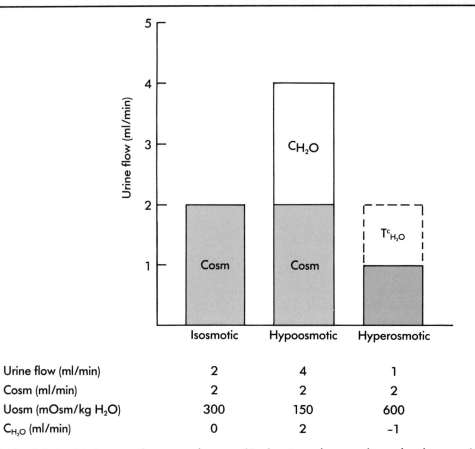

Urine flow (ml/min)	2	4	1
Cosm (ml/min)	2	2	2
Uosm (mOsm/kg H$_2$O)	300	150	600
C$_{H_2O}$ (ml/min)	0	2	-1

Figure 5-10 ■ Relationship between free-water clearance (C$_{H_2O}$), urine volume, and osmolar clearance (C$_{osm}$). With isosmotic urine, there is neither excretion nor reabsorption of solute-free water (C$_{H_2O}$ = 0), and urine flow rate equals C$_{osm}$. With hyposmotic urine, the urine is divided into two virtual volumes; one that contains solute and is isotonic to plasma (urine flow rate = C$_{osm}$), and a volume that is solute-free water (C$_{H_2O}$). With hyperosmotic urine, T$^c_{H_2O}$ (−C$_{H_2O}$) represents the volume of solute-free water that would have to be added to the urine in order to render it isosmotic to plasma.

The clearance of total solute from plasma by the kidneys can be calculated as:

$$C_{osm} = \frac{U_{osm} \times \dot{V}}{P_{osm}} \quad \text{(5-1)}$$

where: C$_{osm}$ is the *osmolar clearance*; U$_{osm}$ is the urine osmolality; $\dot{V}$ is the urine flow rate; and P$_{osm}$ is the plasma osmolality. C$_{osm}$ has units of volume/unit time.

Consider a situation in which the kidneys must excrete 300 mOsm of solute. This can be accomplished by producing urine that is either isosmotic (U$_{osm}$/P$_{osm}$ = 1), hyposmotic (U$_{osm}$/P$_{osm}$<1), or hyperosmotic (U$_{osm}$/P$_{osm}$>1) with respect to plasma. We will examine each of these conditions separately (Figure 5-10).

Example #1—Isosmotic Urine If the urine flow rate under this condition is 2 ml/min, C$_{osm}$ is calculated as:

$$C_{osm} = \frac{300 \text{ mOsm/kg H}_2\text{O} \times 2 \text{ ml/min}}{300 \text{ mOsm/kg H}_2\text{O}} \quad \text{(5-2)}$$

$$= 2 \text{ ml/min}$$

Note that the urine flow rate ($\dot{V}$) is equal to C_{osm}. The significance of this will be explained after considering a situation in which the 300 mOsm of solute is excreted in a dilute urine.

Example #2—Dilute Urine In this situation, the 300 mOsm of solute is excreted in twice the volume. Thus, $U_{osm} = 150$ mOsm/kg H_2O, and $\dot{V} = 4$ ml/min. Accordingly, C_{osm} is calculated as:

$$C_{osm} = \frac{150 \text{ mOsm/kg } H_2O \times 4 \text{ ml/min}}{300 \text{ mOsm/kg } H_2O} \quad (5\text{-}3)$$
$$= 2 \text{ ml/min}$$

Note that C_{osm} is unchanged, but $\dot{V}$ now exceeds it. The difference between these two values represents the solute-free water excreted by the kidneys and is termed the *free-water clearance* (C_{H_2O}). C_{H_2O} is calculated by the following formula:

$$C_{H_2O} = \dot{V} - C_{osm} \quad (5\text{-}4)$$

Equation 5-4 can be expressed in the following way: *Total urine output ($\dot{V}$) consists of two hypothetical components. The first contains all of the solute in a volume that has an osmolality equal to that of plasma (i.e., $U_{osm}/P_{osm} = 1$) and represents a volume from which there has been no separation of solute and water. The second is a volume of solute-free water, defined as C_{H_2O}.*

For the conditions described above:

$$C_{H_2O} = 4 \text{ ml/min} - 2 \text{ ml/min} = 2 \text{ ml/min} \quad (5\text{-}5)$$

For the conditions described in Example #1 (isosmotic urine), the C_{H_2O} is calculated as:

$$C_{H_2O} = 2 \text{ ml/min} - 2 \text{ ml/min} = 0 \quad (5\text{-}6)$$

Thus, with isosmotic urine, there is no excretion of solute-free water.

Example #3—Concentrated Urine In this situation, the 300 mOsm of solute is excreted in half the urine volume. Thus, $U_{osm} = 600$ mOsm/kg H_2O, and $\dot{V} = 1$ ml/min. C_{osm} is calculated as:

$$C_{osm} = \frac{600 \text{ mOsm/kg } H_2O \times 1 \text{ ml/min}}{300 \text{ mOsm/kg } H_2O} \quad (5\text{-}7)$$
$$= 2 \text{ ml/min}$$

Note that C_{osm} is again unchanged. However, $\dot{V}$ is now less than C_{osm}. The difference between these parameters (1 ml/min) represents the solute-free water reabsorbed by the kidneys and returned to systemic circulation.

$$C_{H_2O} = 1 \text{ ml/min} - 2 \text{ ml/min} = -1 \text{ ml/min} \quad (5\text{-}8)$$

By convention, negative C_{H_2O} values are expressed as $T^c_{H_2O}$ (tubular conservation of water). In keeping with the analogy of the situation in which dilute urine was produced, the situation seen with the excretion of concentrated urine can be expressed in the following way: *$T^c_{H_2O}$ represents the volume of water that would have to be added to the urine to reduce its osmolality to a value equal to that of plasma. This represents the volume of solute-free water added to systemic circulation.*

Two points regarding the above examples require emphasis. First, changes in free-water excretion and/or reabsorption occur without changes in solute excretion (C_{osm} is unchanged). This underscores the fact that the control of water balance by the kidneys is independent of the control of excretion of other solutes. Second, C_{H_2O} and $T^c_{H_2O}$ reflect net processes within the kidneys. For example, if C_{H_2O} is equal to zero, there is no net separation of solute and water by the kidneys. In actuality, solute and water were separated by the ascending limb of Henle's loop. However, this solute-free water was reabsorbed by the collecting duct (i.e., solute and water recombined) instead of being excreted (i.e., as dilute urine). The net effect is that C_{H_2O} is zero.

The determination of C_{H_2O} and $T^c_{H_2O}$ can provide important information about the function of those portions of the nephron involved in producing dilute and concentrated urine. Whether the kidneys excrete or reabsorb free water depends upon the presence of ADH.

When no ADH is present or levels are low, solute-free water is excreted. When ADH levels are high, solute-free water is reabsorbed. The magnitude of C_{H_2O} and $T^c_{H_2O}$ vary from individual to individual and are dependent upon a number of factors.

The following factors are necessary for the kidneys to be able to excrete maximally solute-free water (C_{H_2O}):

1. ADH must be absent. This prevents water reabsorption by the collecting duct.
2. The tubular structures, which can separate solute from water (i.e., dilute the luminal fluid), must function normally. In the absence of ADH, the following nephron segments can dilute the luminal fluid:
   a. Ascending thin limb of Henle's loop
   b. Thick ascending limb of Henle's loop
   c. Distal tubule
   d. Collecting duct

   Because of its high transport rate, the thick ascending limb is quantitatively the most important of these segments involved in the separation of solute and water.
3. Adequate delivery of tubular fluid to the above nephron sites is required for maximal separation of solute and water. Factors that reduce delivery (e.g., decreased GFR or enhanced proximal tubule reabsorption) impair the ability of the kidneys to maximally excrete C_{H_2O}.

In the normal adult, the maximum value of C_{H_2O} can be estimated at 10% of the glomerular filtration rate. Thus, if GFR is 180 L/day, the maximum C_{H_2O} is 18 L/day. Under appropriate conditions, an individual could ingest 18 L of water over a 24-hour period, and the kidneys would be able to excrete this as solute-free water. In doing so, the osmolality of the body fluids would be maintained at a normal level. If, however, water intake exceeded 18 L, body fluid osmolality would fall.

The following are required for the kidneys to maximally reabsorb solute-free water ($T^c_{H_2O}$):

1. ADH must be present to allow water reabsorption by the collecting duct. The collecting duct must also be responsive to ADH.
2. The thin and thick ascending limbs of Henle's loop, important to the establishment of the hyperosmotic medullary interstitium, must function normally. Again, because of its high transport capacity, the thick ascending limb is quantitatively the more important segment.
3. A hyperosmotic medullary interstitium is needed to allow water reabsorption by the collecting duct.
4. Adequate delivery of fluid to the ascending limb of Henle's loop is necessary, because the separation of solute and water at this site is needed to maintain the hyperosmotic medullary interstitium.

In the normal adult, $T^c_{H_2O}$ has a maximal value of approximately 8 L/day. Thus, if water loss from other sources (e.g., respiration, perspiration, and in feces) is 1.2 L/day, an individual can go for approximately six to seven days without water and without a rise in plasma osmolality.

■ KEY WORDS AND CONCEPTS

- Antidiuretic hormone (ADH)
- Diuresis/antidiuresis
- Supraoptic nuclei and paraventricular nuclei
- Neurohypophysis/posterior pituitary
- Osmotic and hemodynamic control of ADH secretion
- Osmoreceptors
- Effective and ineffective osmoles
- Set point for osmotic control of ADH secretion
- Baroreceptors
- Cellular events associated with ADH stimulation of collecting duct water permeability
- Polyuria
- Polydipsia
- Diabetes insipidus (central and nephrogenic)

- Syndrome of inappropriate secretion of ADH (SIADH)
- Thirst
- Countercurrent multiplication by Henle's loop
- Single effect of separating solute and water
- Countercurrent exchange by the vasa recta
- Diluting segment (thick ascending limb of Henle's loop)
- Medullary interstitial osmotic gradient
- Medullary accumulation of urea
- Solute-free water
- Free-water clearance (C_{H_2O})
- Free-water reabsorption ($T^c_{H_2O}$)
- Osmolar clearance

■ **SELF-STUDY PROBLEMS**

1. An individual's blood is drawn, and the following values are obtained (normal values are indicated in parenthesis):

Serum [Na$^+$]	135 mEq/L	(140 to 145 mEq/L)
Serum [glucose]	100 mg/dl	(90 to 100 mg/dl)
Serum [urea]	100 mg/dl	(5 to 20 mg/dl)
P_{osm}	310 mOsm/ kg H$_2$O	(285 to 295 mOsm/ kg H$_2$O)

Should plasma ADH levels in this individual be elevated or suppressed?

2. On the table below, indicate the expected osmolality of tubular fluid in the absence and presence of ADH (assume plasma osmolality is 300 mOsm/kg H$_2$O, and osmolality of the medullary interstitium is 1,200 mOsm/kg H$_2$O at the papilla).

3. Given the following data, calculate the free-water excreted by the kidneys.

a. P_{osm} = 295 mOsm/kg H$_2$O
   U_{osm} = 70 mOsm/kg H$_2$O
   $\dot{V}$ = 3 ml/min

b. P_{osm} = 295 mOsm/kg H$_2$O
   U_{osm} = 1,100 mOsm/kg H$_2$O
   $\dot{V}$ = 0.4 ml/min

4. The ability of the kidneys to maximally concentrate the urine is impaired by each of the following conditions:
a. Decreased renal perfusion (i.e., decreased GFR)
b. Administration of a diuretic that inhibits active NaCl transport by the thick ascending limb of Henle's loop
c. Nephrogenic diabetes insipidus
   What are the mechanisms responsible for im-

Nephron site	0-ADH	Max. ADH
Proximal tubule	——	——
Beginning of descending thin limb	——	——
Beginning of ascending thin limb	——	——
End of thick ascending limb	——	——
End of cortical collecting duct	——	——
Urine	——	——

pairment in the kidneys' concentrating ability during each of these conditions?

5. An individual must excrete 800 mOsm of solute in a 24-hour period. What volume of urine is required if the individual can only concentrate the urine to 400 mOsm/kg H_2O? What volume of urine is required if this individual can concentrate the urine to 1,200 mOsm/kg H_2O?

6 Regulation of Extracellular Fluid Volume

■ OBJECTIVES

1. Recognize the vital role Na^+ plays in determining the volume of the extracellular fluid compartment.
2. Explain the concept of "effective circulating volume" and its role in the regulation of renal Na^+ excretion.
3. Describe the mechanisms by which the body monitors the effective circulating volume (volume receptors).
4. Identify the major signals acting on the kidneys to alter their excretion of Na^+.
5. Describe the regulation of Na^+ reabsorption in each of the various portions of the nephron and how changes in effective circulating volume affect these regulatory mechanisms.
6. Explain the pathophysiology of edema formation and the role of Na^+ retention by the kidneys.

The major solutes in extracellular fluid (ECF) are the salts of Na^+. Of these, NaCl is the most abundant and therefore the most important. Since Na^+ (with its salts) is the major determinant of ECF osmolality, it is often assumed that alterations in Na^+ balance result in disturbances in ECF osmolality. However, under normal conditions, this is not the case. The reason for this relates to the presence and sensitivity of the ADH secretory mechanism and thirst, and their roles in regulating water balance. For example, if NaCl was added to the ECF without H_2O, both the $[Na^+]$ and ECF osmolality would increase. The increase in osmolality would stimulate thirst and the release of ADH from the posterior pituitary. The increased ingestion of water in response to thirst, together with the ADH-induced decrease in water excretion by the kidneys, would restore ECF osmolality to normal. However, the volume of the ECF would be increased in proportion to the amount of water ingested, which in turn is dependent upon the amount of NaCl added to the ECF. Conversely, a decrease in the NaCl content of the ECF will result in a decrease in the volume of this compartment. Thus, provided the ADH and thirst sytems are functioning normally, alterations in the NaCl content of the ECF result in parallel changes in ECF volume.

The kidneys are the major route for excretion of NaCl from the body. As such, they play an important role in regulating the volume of the ECF. Under normal conditions, the kidneys keep the volume of the ECF constant by adjusting the excretion of NaCl to match the amount ingested in the diet. If ingestion exceeds excretion, ECF volume increases above normal, whereas the opposite occurs if excretion exceeds ingestion.

To defend itself against changes in ECF volume, the body relies on a system that monitors the volume of this compartment and sends signals to the kidneys to make appropriate adjustments in NaCl excretion.

This chapter reviews the physiology of the volume receptors and explains the signals that act on the kidneys to regulate NaCl excretion, along with the responses of the various portions of the nephron to these signals. In addition, the pathophysiological mechanisms involved in the formation of edema are presented, with emphasis on the handling of NaCl by the kidneys.

■ CONCEPT OF EFFECTIVE CIRCULATING VOLUME

To understand the role of the kidneys in regulating ECF volume, it is necessary to consider the concept of *effective circulating volume (ECV)*. ECV is not a measurable and distinct body fluid compartment; rather, it is related to the adequacy of tissue perfusion. Thus, it is related to the "fullness" of and "pressure" within the vascular tree. In the normal individual, ECV varies in parallel to the volume of the ECF. However, this relationship is not maintained under some pathological conditions. For example, in patients with heart disease, ECV can be reduced due to reduced cardiac output, yet the volume of the ECF may be increased above normal.

An important point regarding ECV is that the kidneys will alter their excretion of NaCl in response to changes in this parameter. When ECV is decreased, renal NaCl excretion is reduced. This adaptive response restores ECV to its normal value and maintains adequate tissue perfusion. Conversely, an increase in ECV results in enhanced renal NaCl excretion, termed *natriuresis*. Figure 6-1 illustrates the components of the ECV regulatory system, each of which is discussed in detail below.

In the normal individual, the terms ECV and ECF can be, and often are, interchanged. However, it is the ECV, especially under certain pathological conditions, that determines renal Na^+ excretion. Consequently, to provide a framework for understanding the pathophysiological basis of some clinically significant conditions, the remaining sections of this chapter will refer primarily to the ECV.

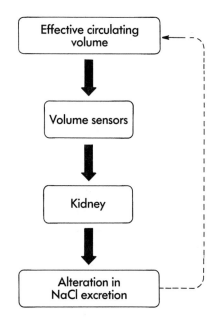

Figure 6-1 ■ General scheme for monitoring and controlling the effective circulating volume.

ECV volume receptors

Vascular
    Low pressure
        Cardiac atria
        Pulmonary vasculature
    High pressure
        Carotid sinus
        Aortic arch
        Juxtaglomerular apparatus of kidney
           (afferent arteriole)
Central nervous system
Hepatic

■ ECV VOLUME SENSORS

The various volume sensors in the body are listed in the box on p. 92. Sensors have been identified in the vascular tree, where they monitor its fullness and pressure. These vascular volume receptors appear to be the primary sensors for ECV. Receptors related to the control of NaCl excretion by the kidneys are also assumed to exist within the brain and liver. Less is known about these latter two groups of receptors, and are not considered further in this text. The receptors in the vascular system respond to stretch *(baroreceptors)* and are considered in more detail below.

Vascular Low-Pressure Volume Receptors

Baroreceptors are located within the walls of the cardiac atria and pulmonary vessels, and respond to distention of these structures. Because of the low pressure within the atria and pulmonary vessels, these receptors respond primarily to the "fullness" of the vascular tree, sending signals to the brain's hypothalamic and medullary regions via afferent fibers in the vagus nerve. (Distention results in an increase in the number of impulses per second.) In response to this vagal input, sympathetic outflow from the central nervous system and secretion of ADH by the posterior pituitary are altered.

The cardiac atria possess an additional mechanism for the control of renal NaCl excretion and thus ECV. The myocytes of the atria synthesize and store a peptide hormone. This hormone, termed *atrial natriuretic peptide (ANP)*, is released when the atria are distended (i.e., expansion of the ECV) and, by the mechanisms outlined in subsequent sections, rapidly increases the excretion of NaCl and water by the kidneys.

Vascular High-Pressure Volume Receptors

Baroreceptors are also present in the arterial side of the vascular tree, located in the wall of the aortic arch, the carotid sinus, and the affer-ent arteriole of the kidneys. These receptors respond primarily to blood pressure. The aortic arch and carotid baroreceptors, like the low-pressure receptors, send input to the hypothalamic and medullary centers of the brain via the vagus and glossopharyngeal nerves. (Increased arterial pressure leads to an increase in the number of impulses per second.) The response to this input also involves alterations in sympathetic outflow from the CNS and ADH secretion by the posterior pituitary.

The *juxtaglomerular apparatus* (see Chapter 2), particularly the afferent arteriole of the glomerulus, acts as a high-pressure baroreceptor. Changes in perfusion pressure at this site lead to alterations in renin secretion. Renin in turn determines the levels of angiotensin II and aldosterone, both of which play an important role in regulating renal Na^+ excretion.

■ VOLUME RECEPTOR SIGNALS

Once the volume receptors have detected a change in the ECV, they send signals to the kidneys, which result in an appropriate adjustment of NaCl and water excretion. Both neural and hormonal signals have been identified. These signals are summarized in the box on page 94, as are their effects on renal NaCl and water excretion.

Renal Sympathetic Nerves

As described in Chapter 2, *sympathetic nerve* fibers innervate the afferent and efferent arterioles of the glomerulus, as well as nephron cells. When ECV is decreased, decreased afferent input to the CNS from the low and high pressure baroreceptors results in increased renal sympathetic nerve activity. This has the following effects:

1. The afferent and efferent arterioles are constricted. This vasoconstriction (the effect appears to be greater on the afferent arteriole) decreases the volume of plasma flowing through the glomerulus and the hydrostatic

---

> ### *Signals involved in the control of renal NaCl and water excretion*
>
> **Renal Sympathetic Nerves (↑ Activity: ↓ NaCl Excretion)**
>
> - ↓ Glomerular filtration rate
> - ↑ Renin secretion
> - ↑ Proximal tubule and thick ascending limb of Henle's loop NaCl reabsorption
>
> **Renin-Angiotensin-Aldosterone (↑ Secretion: ↓ NaCl Excretion)**
>
> - ↑ Angiotensin II levels stimulate proximal tubule NaCl reabsorption
> - ↑ Aldosterone levels stimulate thick ascending limb of Henle's loop and collecting duct NaCl reabsorption
> - ↑ ADH secretion
>
> **Atrial Natriuretic Peptide (↑ Secretion: ↑ NaCl Excretion)**
>
> - ↑ Glomerular filtration rate
> - ↓ Renin secretion
> - ↓ Aldosterone secretion
> - ↓ NaCl reabsorption by the collecting duct
> - ↓ ADH secretion
>
> **ADH (↑ Secretion: ↓ H_2O and NaCl Excretion)**
>
> - ↑ H_2O absorption by the collecting duct
> - ↑ NaCl reabsorption by the thick ascending limb of Henle's loop
> - ↑ NaCl reabsorption by the collecting duct

pressure within the glomerular capillary lumen. The net effect of these changes in glomerular hemodynamics is a reduction in the glomerular filtration rate. With this decrease in GFR, the filtered load of Na^+ is reduced (filtered load = GFR $\times$ plasma $[Na^+]$).

2. Renin secretion by the cells of the afferent and efferent arterioles is stimulated. As described below, renin leads to increased circulating levels of angiotensin II and aldosterone.

3. NaCl reabsorption by the proximal tubule and Henle's loop is directly stimulated.

The combined effect of these actions contributes to an overall decrease in NaCl excretion, an adaptive response that works to restore ECV to its normal value.

When the volume of ECV is increased, renal sympathetic nerve activity is reduced. This generally reverses the effects described above.

Renin-Angiotensin-Aldosterone System

Smooth muscle cells in the afferent and efferent arterioles of the glomerulus are the site of synthesis, storage, and release of renin. Three factors play an important role in stimulating renin secretion:

1. Perfusion pressure—The afferent arteriole behaves as a high-pressure baroreceptor. When perfusion pressure to the kidneys is reduced, renin secretion is stimulated. Conversely, an increase in perfusion pressure inhibits renin release.

2. Sympathetic nerve activity—Activation of the sympathetic nerve fibers innervating the afferent and efferent arterioles results in an increase in renin secretion. Renin secretion is decreased as renal sympathetic nerve activity is decreased.

3. Delivery of NaCl to the macula densa—Delivery of NaCl to the macula densa regulates the GFR (see Chapter 4). With increased delivery, GFR decreases, and decreased delivery increases GFR. In addition, renin secretion is altered. When NaCl delivery is decreased, renin secretion is enhanced. Conversely, an increase in NaCl delivery inhibits renin secretion.

Figure 6-2 summarizes the essential components of the renin-angiotensin-aldosterone system. Renin alone does not directly alter renal function. It is a proteolytic enzyme, and its substrate is a circulating peptide (angiotensinogen), which is produced by the liver. *Angiotensinogen* is cleaved by renin to a 10-amino acid

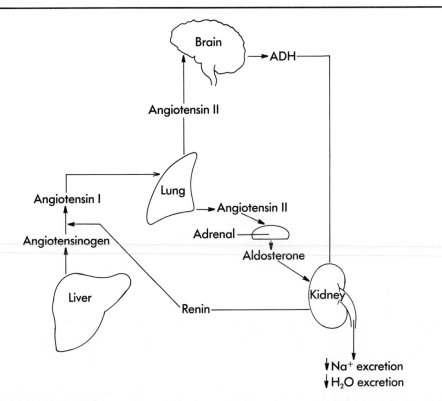

Figure 6-2 ■ Schematic representation of the essential components of the renin-angiotensin-aldosterone system. Activation of this system results in a decrease in the excretion of Na⁺ and water. See text for details.

peptide *(angiotensin I)*. Angiotensin I, like renin, does not appear to have a direct effect on the kidneys. It is cleaved to an 8-amino acid peptide (angiotensin II), by a *converting enzyme*. This enzyme is found in high concentrations in the lung. Nearly all angiotensin I is converted to angiotensin II in a single pass through the pulmonary circulation. Angiotensin II acts as a negative feedback regulator of renin secretion (i.e., inhibits renin secretion) and has the following important physiological functions:

1. Stimulation of aldosterone secretion by glomerulosa cells of the adrenal cortex.
2. Vasoconstriction of capillary arterioles, which increases blood pressure.
3. Stimulation of ADH secretion from the pos-

terior pituitary and stimulation of the thirst center within the hypothalamus.
4. Enhancement of NaCl reabsorption by the proximal tubule.

Angiotensin II is an important secretagogue for aldosterone; a steroid hormone produced by the glomerulosa cells of the adrenal cortex. Aldosterone acts in a number of ways on the kidneys (see Chapters 4, 7, and 8). With regard to the regulation of ECV, aldosterone reduces NaCl excretion by stimulating its reabsorption by the thick ascending limb of Henle's loop, the distal tubule, and collecting duct.

Aldosterone stimulation of Na⁺ reabsorption in the late portion of the distal tubule and collecting duct has been studied extensively. In

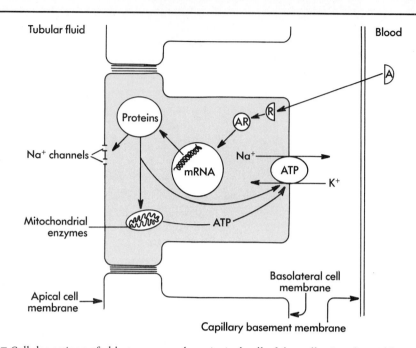

Tubular fluid

Blood

Proteins

AR

R

A

Na⁺ channels

I

mRNA

Na⁺

ATP

K⁺

Mitochondrial enzymes

ATP

Apical cell membrane

Basolateral cell membrane

Capillary basement membrane

Figure 6-3 ■ Cellular actions of aldosterone on the principal cell of the collecting duct. Aldosterone *(A)* binds to an intracellular receptor *(R)*. The receptor-aldosterone complex *(AR)* regulates the transcription of specific mRNA, and ultimately the synthesis of proteins. It is postulated that these aldosterone-induced proteins include apical membrane Na⁺ channels, mitochondrial enzymes, and the Na⁺-K⁺-ATPase. As a result of aldosterone's actions reabsorption of Na⁺ from the tubular fluid is increased.

these segments, aldosterone stimulates Na⁺ reabsorption by the principal cell (Figure 6-3). Aldosterone enters the cell and binds to a cytoplasmic receptor. The hormone-receptor complex interacts with specific binding sites on deoxyribonucleic acid (DNA), thereby regulating the transcription of messenger ribonucleic acid (mRNA). Translation of these messages results in increased levels of a number of proteins important to Na⁺ reabsorption by the cell. It has been postulated that these *aldosterone-induced proteins* include new apical membrane Na⁺ channels, enzymes necessary for the synthesis of adenosine triphosphate (ATP), and Na⁺-K⁺-ATPase.

By these actions, Na⁺ entry into the cell across the apical membrane is enhanced, as is its extrusion from the cell across the basolateral

membrane. Because Na⁺ reabsorption generates a lumen negative transepithelial voltage (see Chapter 4), the enhanced Na⁺ reabsorption from the luminal fluid increases the magnitude of this voltage. The passive movement of Cl⁻ from the lumen to blood via the paracellular pathway is enhanced by this voltage change. Thus, aldosterone increases the reabsorption of NaCl from the tubular fluid. Reduced levels of aldosterone result in a decrease in the amount of NaCl reabsorbed by the principal cell.

Aldosterone also enhances NaCl reabsorption by cells of the thick ascending limb of Henle's loop, although the precise cellular mechanisms involved have not yet been elucidated.

In general, activation of the renin-angiotensin-aldosterone system results in decreased NaCl excretion by the kidneys. This system is suppressed when ECV is expanded, and renal NaCl excretion is therefore enhanced.

Atrial Natriuretic Peptide

Atrial myocytes produce and store a peptide hormone, called *atrial natriuretic peptide (ANP)*, that promotes NaCl and water excretion by the kidneys. ANP is released with atrial stretch, as would occur with expansion of the ECV. The circulating form of ANP is 28 amino acids in length. In general, its actions antagonize those of the renin-angiotensin-aldosterone system. They include the following:

1. Vasodilation of the afferent and efferent arterioles of the glomerulus, increasing renal plasma flow and GFR (with an increase in GFR, the filtered load of Na^+ is increased)*.
2. Inhibition of renin secretion by the afferent and efferent arterioles.
3. Aldosterone secretion by the glomerulosa cells of the adrenal cortex is inhibited. ANP reduces aldosterone secretion by two mechanisms: Angiotensin II-induced aldosterone secretion is reduced secondary to ANP inhibition of renin secretion, and ANP acts directly on the glomerulosa cells of the adrenal cortex to inhibit aldosterone secretion.
4. NaCl reabsorption by the collecting duct is inhibited. This is due in part to reduced levels of aldosterone; however, ANP also acts directly on the collecting duct cells. Through its second-messenger cyclic guanine monophosphate (cGMP), ANP inhibits NaCl reabsorption. This effect is predominantly in the medullary portion of the collecting duct.
5. ADH secretion by the posterior pituitary and ADH action on the collecting duct are inhibited. This results in a reduction of water reabsorption by the collecting duct and thus increased excretion of water in the urine.

ANP is also an important vasodilator, which explains the reduction in blood pressure seen with ANP.

Taken together, these effects of ANP increase excretion of NaCl and water. Hypothetically, a reduction in circulating levels of ANP would be expected to decrease NaCl and water excretion. However, there is no convincing evidence in this regard.

Antidiuretic Hormone

When ECV is reduced, and in response to decreased baroreceptor input, ADH secretion by the posterior pituitary is stimulated. ADH increases the water permeability of the collecting duct and enhances NaCl reabsorption by the thick ascending limb of Henle's loop and the collecting duct. Thus, NaCl and water excretion is reduced to restore ECV to normal levels. An increase in ECV reduces ADH secretion in response to increased baroreceptor input and contributes to the associated increase in NaCl and water excretion.

■ CONTROL OF Na^+ EXCRETION WITH NORMAL ECV

The maintenance of a normal ECV, termed *euvolemia*, requires the precise balance between the amount of NaCl ingested and that excreted from the body.* Because the kidneys are the major route for NaCl excretion, the amount of NaCl in the urine will reflect dietary intake. Thus, *in a euvolemic individual, daily urine NaCl excretion equals daily NaCl intake.*

The kidneys can vary the amount of NaCl they excrete over a wide range. Under conditions of NaCl restriction (i.e., low NaCl diet), virtually no NaCl appears in the urine. Conversely, in individuals who ingest large quantities of NaCl, renal excretion can exceed 1,000 mEq/day. The

---

*Because GFR is increased, the effect of ANP on the afferent arteriole must predominate.

*During euvolemia, the ECV varies in direct proportion to the volume of the ECF. Thus, the two terms can be interchanged.

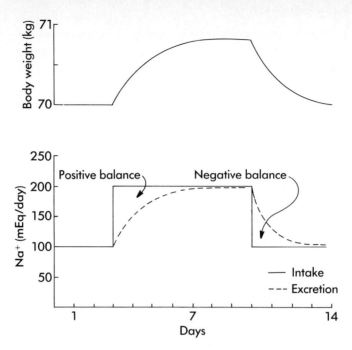

Figure 6-4 ▪ Response to step increases and decreases in NaCl intake. NaCl excretion lags behind abrupt changes in NaCl intake. The change in extracellular fluid volume is sensed by the volume receptors, and leads to appropriate adjustments in the renal NaCl excretion. The transient periods of positive and negative balance result in alterations in the volume of the extracellular fluid, which are detected as changes in body weight.

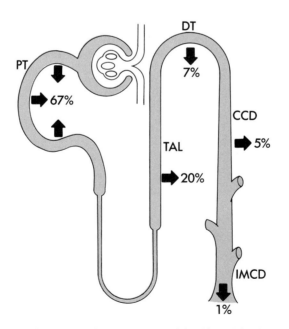

Figure 6-5 ▪ Segmental Na$^+$ reabsorption. The percentage of the filtered load of Na$^+$ reabsorbed by each nephron segment is indicated. *PT*, proximal tubule; *TAL*, thick ascending limb; *DT*, distal tubule; *CCD*, cortical collecting duct; *IMCD*, inner medullary collecting duct.

kidneys' response to variations in dietary NaCl usually takes several days. This is especially true when significant changes occur. During the transition period, excretion does not match intake, and the individual will either be in a *positive* (intake > excretion) or *negative* (intake < excretion) *NaCl balance.*

In the example shown in Figure 6-4, NaCl intake is abruptly increased. During the transition period required for the kidney to increase its excretion, a state of positive balance exists. The retained NaCl is added to the extracellular fluid, which increases in volume (water via the ADH system is also retained to keep plasma osmolality constant). The individual can detect this increase in ECF volume by a gain in body weight (1 L of ECF ≅ 1 kg). Note that after several days excretion again equals intake, but at a higher level. When the intake is abruptly returned to its original level, a period of negative balance exists; however, after a few days excretion again equals intake. Body weight also returns to its original level, reflecting the decrease in ECF volume.

To understand how renal NaCl is regulated, the general features of Na^+ handling along the nephron must be clear. Figure 6-5 summarizes the contribution of each nephron segment to the reabsorption of the filtered load of Na^+ under euvolemic conditions (the specific cellular mechanisms of Na^+ transport are explained in Chapter 4). Although there is parallel reabsorption of Cl^-, this discussion only addresses Na^+ reabsorption.

In a normal adult, the filtered load of Na^+ can be calculated as:

$$\text{Filtered load of } Na^+ = (GFR)(\text{plasma }[Na^+]) \qquad (6\text{-}1)$$
$$= (180 \text{ L/day})(140 \text{ mEq/L})$$
$$= 25,200 \text{ mEq/day}$$

With a typical diet, only about 1% or less of this filtered load is excreted in the urine (<250 mEq/day). It is important to recognize that, because of the large filtered load of Na^+, small changes in Na^+ reabsorption by the nephron can have a large effect on Na^+ balance and thus ECF volume. For example, an increase in Na^+ excretion from 1% to 3% of the filtered load represents an additional loss of approximately 500 mEq/day. Because the ECF $[Na^+]$ is 140 mEq/L, Na^+ loss of this magnitude would decrease ECF volume by more than 3 L (500 mEq/day/140 mEq/L = 3.6 L).

Regulation of renal Na^+ excretion requires the integrated action of all nephron segments. During euvolemia, Na^+ handling by the nephron can be explained by two general processes:

1. *Na^+ reabsorption by the proximal tubule, Henle's loop, and the distal tubule is regulated so that a relatively constant portion of the filtered load of Na^+ is delivered to the collecting duct.* As indicated in Figure 6-5, the combined action of these nephron segments delivers 6% of the filtered load to the beginning of the collecting duct.

2. *Reabsorption of Na^+ by the collecting duct is regulated such that the amount of Na^+ excreted in the urine matches the amount ingested in the diet.* Thus, the collecting duct is the site where final adjustments in Na^+ excretion are made to maintain the euvolemic state.

Mechanisms for Keeping Na^+ Delivery to the Collecting Duct Constant

A number of mechanisms maintain delivery of a constant fraction of the filtered load of Na^+ to the beginning of the collecting duct. These are autoregulation of GFR, and thus the filtered load of Na^+; glomerulotubular balance; and load dependency of Na^+ reabsorption by Henle's loop and the distal tubule.

Autoregulation of GFR (see Chapter 3), allows for the maintenance of a relatively constant filtration rate over a wide range of perfusion pressures. Because of this constant filtration rate, the filtered load of Na^+ is also kept constant.

Despite the autoregulatory control of GFR, small variations occur. If these changes were not compensated for by an appropriate adjustment in Na$^+$ reabsorption by the nephron, marked changes in Na$^+$ excretion would result. However, Na$^+$ reabsorption, especially by the proximal tubule, does change parallel to changes in GFR, a phenomenon termed *glomerulotubular balance (GT-balance)*. By this process, reabsorption of Na$^+$, primarily by the proximal tubule, is adjusted to match the GFR. Thus, if GFR increases, the amount of Na$^+$ reabsorbed by this nephron segment also increases. The opposite occurs if GFR decreases. (GT-balance is further described in Chapter 4.)

The final mechanism that contributes to the constant delivery of Na$^+$ to the beginning of the collecting duct relates to the ability of Henle's loop and the distal tubule to increase their Na$^+$ reabsorptive rates in response to an increase in delivery. Of these two segments, Henle's loop, particularly the thick ascending limb, has the greater capacity to increase Na$^+$ reabsorption in response to increased delivery. The mechanism responsible for this likely reflects the fact that, under normal conditions, the transport capacity for these segments is not saturated. Thus, an increase in delivery is simply compensated for by an increase in reabsorption.

Regulation of Collecting Duct Na$^+$ Reabsorption

With a constant delivery of Na$^+$, small adjustments in collecting duct reabsorption are sufficient to balance excretion with intake. (Recall that a 2% change in the fractional excretion of Na$^+$ represents more than 3 L of ECF.) Aldosterone is the primary regulator of collecting duct Na$^+$ reabsorption and thus Na$^+$ excretion under this condition. When aldosterone levels are elevated, Na$^+$ reabsorption by the collecting duct is increased (excretion decreased), while Na$^+$ reabsorption is decreased (excretion increased) when aldosterone levels are suppressed.

A number of other hormones alter collecting duct Na$^+$ reabsorption, including ANP, prostaglandins, and bradykinin. ADH, in addition to enhancing water reabsorption by the collecting duct, stimulates Na$^+$ reabsorption. However, at present, the relative roles of these other hormones in the regulation of collecting duct Na$^+$ reabsorption during euvolemia are not clear.

As long as variations in the dietary intake of NaCl are minor, the mechanisms described above can regulate Na$^+$ excretion appropriately, thereby maintaining ECV volume at a normal level. However, significant changes in NaCl intake cannot be handled effectively by these mechanisms, and ECV is altered. When this occurs, additional factors are called into play that act on the kidneys to adjust Na$^+$ reabsorption and reestablish the euvolemic state.

■ CONTROL OF Na$^+$ EXCRETION WITH INCREASED ECV

An above normal increase in ECV is detected by the volume sensors, and signals are sent to the kidneys, resulting in an increase in Na$^+$ excretion. The signals acting on the kidneys include:

1. Decreased activity of the renal sympathetic nerves.
2. Release of ANP from atrial myocytes.
3. Inhibition of ADH secretion by the posterior pituitary.
4. Decreased renin secretion, and thus decreased angiotensin II production and decreased aldosterone secretion by the adrenal cortex.

The integrated response of the nephron to these signals is illustrated in Figure 6-6. *The important difference between the situation of an above-normal increase in ECV and that of the euvolemic state is that the renal response is not limited to the collecting duct; rather, it involves the entire nephron.*

Three general responses to an increase in ECV occur (Figure 6-6):

1. *GFR increases*—GFR increases primarily

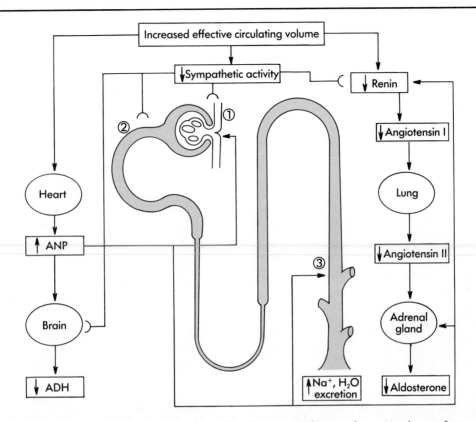

Figure 6-6 ■ Integrated response to expansion of the effective circulating volume. Numbers refer to description of the response in the text.

as a result of the decrease in sympathetic nerve activity. Sympathetic fibers innervate the afferent and efferent arterioles of the glomerulus and control their diameter. Decreased sympathetic nerve activity leads to their dilation. Because the effect appears to be greater on the afferent arteriole, the hydrostatic pressure within the glomerular capillary increases. Renal plasma flow also increases with dilation of the afferent and efferent arterioles. As a result of these changes in glomerular hemodynamics, GFR increases. ANP has also been shown to increase GFR by dilating the afferent and efferent arterioles. The increased ANP levels found with this condition are also likely to contribute to this

response. With an increase in GFR, the filtered load of Na^+ increases.

2. *Reabsorption of Na^+ decreases in the proximal tubule*—Several mechanisms appear to be involved in reducing Na^+ reabsorption by the proximal tubule, but controversy remains regarding the precise role of each. Because activation of the sympathetic nerve fibers innervating this region stimulates Na^+ reabsorption, the decreased sympathetic nerve activity resulting from increased ECV may contribute to decreased Na^+ reabsorption. In addition, angiotensin II directly stimulates Na^+ reabsorption by the proximal tubule. Because angiotensin II levels are also reduced under this condition, it is possible

that proximal tubule Na$^+$ reabsorption is decreased as a result. With dilation of the afferent and efferent arterioles, the hydrostatic pressure within the peritubular capillaries is increased. This alteration in the Starling forces reduces the absorption of solute (e.g., Na$^+$) and water from the lateral intercellular space, thus reducing tubular reabsorption (see Chapter 4 for mechanism).

3. *Na$^+$ reabsorption decreases in the collecting duct*—Both the increase in filtered load and the decrease in proximal tubule reabsorption result in the delivery of large amounts of NaCl to Henle's loop and the distal convoluted tubule. Because in-

creased activity of sympathetic nerves and aldosterone stimulates NaCl reabsorption by Henle's loop, the reduced nerve activity and low aldosterone levels seen with an expanded ECV could in theory reduce NaCl reabsorption by this nephron segment. However, because reabsorption by the thick ascending limb is load-dependent, these effects are offset, and the fraction of the filtered load of Na$^+$ reabsorbed by Henle's loop is actually increased. Nevertheless, the amount of Na$^+$ delivered to the beginning of the collecting duct is increased compared with the euvolemic state (Figure 6-7).

The amount of Na$^+$ delivered to the begin-

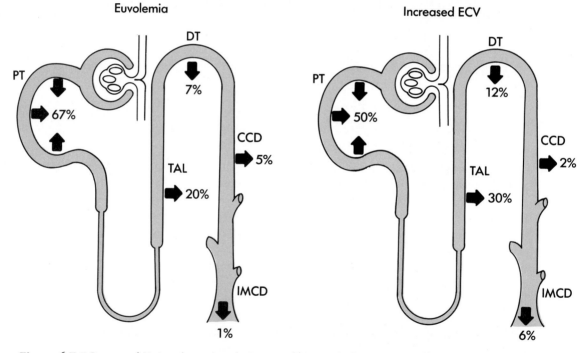

Figure 6-7 ■ Segmental Na$^+$ reabsorption during euvolemia and after expansion of the effective circulating volume (ECV). Note that with expansion of the ECV delivery of Na$^+$ to the collecting duct is increased from 6% to 8%. With inhibition of Na$^+$ reabsorption by the collecting duct Na$^+$ excretion is increased from 1% to 6%. *PT*, proximal tubule; *TAL*, thick ascending limb; *DT*, distal tubule; *CCD*, cortical collecting duct; *IMCD*, inner medullary collecting duct.

ning of the collecting duct varies in proportion to the degree of ECV expansion. A larger load of Na^+ overwhelms the reabsorptive capacity of the collecting duct, which is even further reduced by the actions of ANP and the decrease in the circulating levels of aldosterone.

The final component in the response to ECV expansion is the excretion of water. As Na^+ excretion increases, plasma osmolality begins to fall. This results in decreased secretion of ADH. ADH secretion is also decreased by baroreceptor activity and the action of ANP. In addition, ANP inhibits the action of ADH on the collecting duct. Together, these effects decrease water reabsorption by the collecting duct, thereby increasing water excretion by the kidneys. Thus, the excretion of NaCl and water occurs in concert; ECV is restored to normal, and body fluid osmolality remains constant.

In summary, the nephron's response to ECV expansion involves the integrated action of all of its component parts. The filtered load is increased, proximal tubule reabsorption is reduced (GFR is increased, while proximal reabsorption is decreased; thus, GT-balance does not occur under this condition), and the delivery of Na^+ to the beginning of the collecting duct is increased. This increased delivery, with inhibition of collecting duct reabsorption, results in the excretion of a larger fraction of the filtered load of Na^+. The excretion of Na^+ will exceed intake (negative balance), and the ECV will be restored to normal. The time course of this restoration (hours to days) depends upon the degree to which the ECV is increased above normal and the magnitude of the difference between intake and excretion of Na^+.

■ CONTROL OF Na^+ EXCRETION WITH DECREASED ECV

Volume sensors detect a decrease in ECV. Signals are sent to the kidneys, and Na^+ and water excretion are reduced. The signals involved are essentially the opposite of those involved with

the response to ECV expansion, and include:
1. Increased renal sympathetic nerve activity.
2. Increased secretion of renin, which results in increased angiotensin II levels and thus increased secretion of aldosterone by the adrenal cortex.
3. Inhibition of ANP secretion by the atrial myocytes.
4. Stimulation of ADH secretion by the posterior pituitary.

The integrated response of the nephron to these signals is illustrated in Figure 6-8.

The nephron's response to ECV contraction involves all of the nephron segments. The general response is as follows:
1. *GFR decreases*—Afferent and efferent arteriolar constriction occurs as a result of increased renal sympathetic nerve activity. The effect appears to be greater on the afferent arteriole, causing the hydrostatic pressure in the glomerular capillary to fall. Renal plasma flow also declines. The net effect of these changes in glomerular hemodynamics is a decrease in GFR. This in turn reduces the filtered load of Na^+.
2. *Na^+ reabsorption by the proximal tubule is increased*—Several mechanisms may be involved in augmenting Na^+ reabsorption in this segment. For example, increased sympathetic nerve activity and angiotensin II directly stimulate proximal tubule Na^+ reabsorption. With constriction of the afferent and efferent arterioles, the hydrostatic pressure within the peritubular capillaries is reduced. This facilitates the movement of fluid from the lateral intercellular space into the capillary, thereby stimulating proximal tubule reabsorption of solute and water (see Chapter 4 for mechanism).
3. *Na^+ reabsorption by the collecting duct is enhanced*—The reduction in filtered load and enhanced proximal tubule reabsorption result in decreased delivery of

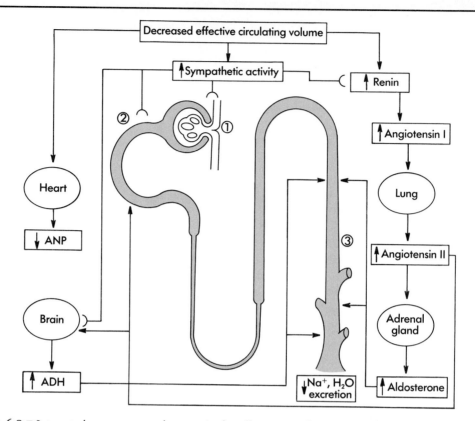

Figure 6-8 ■ Integrated response to a decrease in the effective circulating volume. Numbers refer to description of the response in text.

Na$^+$ to Henle's loop and the distal tubule. Increased sympathetic nerve activity, ADH and aldosterone have been shown to stimulate Na$^+$ reabsorption by the thick ascending limb. Aldosterone and ADH also act on the distal tubule to increase Na$^+$ reabsorption at this site. Because sympathetic nerve activity is increased and ADH and aldosterone levels are elevated with a decreased ECV, the potential for increased Na$^+$ reabsorption by these segments exists. However, Na$^+$ transport by the thick ascending limb and distal tubule is load-dependent. This offsets the stimulatory effects of increased sympathetic nerve activity, ADH, and aldosterone, and the frac-

tion of the filtered load of Na$^+$ reabsorbed by these segments is actually less than that seen in the euvolemic state. Nevertheless, the net result of decreased GFR, together with enhanced proximal tubule reabsorption and additional reabsorption, albeit at reduced rates, by Henle's loop and the distal convoluted tubule is that less Na$^+$ is delivered to the beginning of the collecting duct. This is illustrated in Figure 6-9.

The small amount of Na$^+$ delivered to the collecting duct is virtually all reabsorbed, because transport in this segment is enhanced. This stimulation of collecting duct Na$^+$ reabsorption is primarily due to increased aldosterone levels. Additionally, ANP, which inhibits

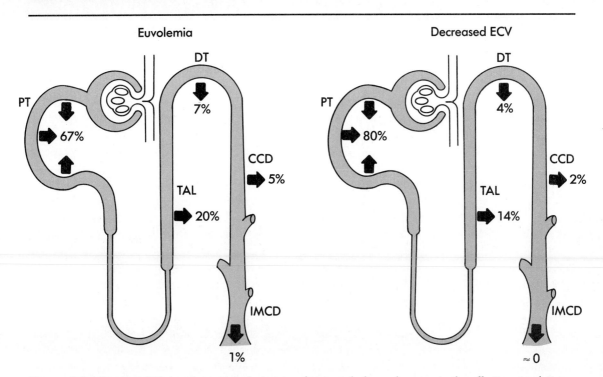

Figure 6-9 ■ Segmental Na^+ reabsorption during euvolemia and after a decrease in the effective circulating volume (ECV). Note that with contraction of the ECV delivery of Na^+ to the collecting duct is reduced from 6% to 2%. The collecting duct reabsorbs virtually all of the Na^+ it receives, and Na^+ excretion is reduced to near zero. *PT*, proximal tubule; *TAL*, thick ascending limb; *DT*, distal tubule; *CCD*, cortical collecting duct; *IMCD*, inner medullary collecting duct.

collecting duct reabsorption, is not present, and ADH, which can stimulate Na^+ reabsorption, is present at high levels.

Finally, water reabsorption by the collecting duct is enhanced by ADH, the levels of which are elevated due to activation of the baroreceptors. As a result, water excretion is reduced and, together with the NaCl retained by the kidneys, ECV is restored and body fluid osmolality remains constant.

In summary, the nephron's response to ECV contraction, like that seen with ECV expansion, involves the integrated action of all of its component segments. The filtered load of Na^+ is decreased, proximal tubule reabsorption is enhanced (GFR is decreased, while proximal reab-

sorption is increased; thus, GT-balance does not occur under this condition), and the delivery of Na^+ to the beginning of the collecting duct is reduced. This decreased delivery, together with enhanced Na^+ reabsorption by the collecting duct, results in the virtual elimination of Na^+ from the urine. Thus, excretion of Na^+ is less than intake (positive balance), and ECV is reexpanded. The time course of this reexpansion (hours to days) depends on the degree to which ECV is reduced from normal and the dietary intake of Na^+.

■ EDEMA AND THE ROLE OF THE KIDNEYS

Edema is the accumulation of excess fluid within the interstitial space. The Starling forces across the capillaries determine the movement of fluid out of the vascular compartment into the interstitial space. Alterations of these forces under pathological conditions can lead to increased movement of fluid from the vascular space into the interstitium, resulting in edema formation. However, in order for edema to be detected clinically (e.g., swelling of ankles), NaCl and water must be retained by the kidneys.

The role of the kidneys in edema formation can be appreciated by recognizing that the interstitial compartment must contain 2 to 3 L of excess fluid before edema is detectable. The source of this fluid is the vascular compartment (i.e., plasma), which has a volume of 3 to 4 L in the normal individual. Thus, the movement of 2 to 3 L out of the plasma compartment into the interstitial compartment would result in a marked decrease in blood pressure. As described below, this would prevent further movement of fluid from the vascular compartment into the interstitial compartment. However, retention of NaCl and water by the kidneys replenishes the plasma volume, thereby maintaining blood pressure. As a result, the accumulation of fluid in the interstitial compartment continues, and edema develops.

Alterations in Starling Forces

In Chapter 1, the Starling forces and their determination of fluid movement across the capillary wall were explained. Considering all capillary beds (exclusive of the glomerulus) under normal conditions, approximately 20 L/day moves out of the capillary at the arteriole end, 18 L/day is absorbed back into the capillary at the venous end, and 2 L/day returns to circulation via the lymphatics. Edema results from a change in the Starling forces that alter these fluid dynamics.

Capillary Hydrostatic Pressure (P_c) Increasing P_c favors the movement of fluid out of the capillary or retards its movement into the capillary, thereby promoting edema formation.

Normally, the resistance of the precapillary arteriole is well-regulated, such that changes in systemic blood pressure do not result in marked alterations in P_c. However, alterations in the pressure within the venous side of circulation do have a significant effect on P_c. Consequently, an increase in venous pressure will elevate P_c. This reduces the amount of fluid reabsorbed from the interstitium back into the capillary lumen, resulting in the accumulation of edema fluid. Heart failure is one of the common conditions producing an increase in P_c. Because of poor cardiac performance, the pressure in the venous circulation is elevated. P_c can also be elevated secondary to venous thrombosis.

Plasma Oncotic Pressure (Π_c) A decrease in Π_c favors movement of fluid out of the capillary lumen and inhibits its reabsorption from the interstitium. Alterations in Π_c result primarily from changes in the plasma [albumin]. With some renal diseases, the permeability of the glomerular capillary is abnormally high, causing large quantities of albumin to be filtered and lost in the urine. If the rate of loss exceeds the rate at which albumin is synthesized by the liver, plasma [albumin] will fall, and edema can form.

Lymphatic Obstruction Obstruction of the lymphatics will interfere with and reduce the volume of interstitial fluid that is returned to circulation via this route. As a result, edema can form. The most common cause of lymphatic obstruction is malignancy; when malignant cells spread to lymph nodes, obstruction can occur.

Capillary Permeability An increase in capillary permeability favors increased movement of fluid across the capillary wall, aiding capillary-to-interstitium movement at the arteriolar end and interstitium-to-capillary movement at the venous end. Because permeability is increased, albumin can accumulate in the interstitium. The oncotic pressure of the albumin will result in the accumulation of excess fluid in the interstitial compartment, and edema will form.

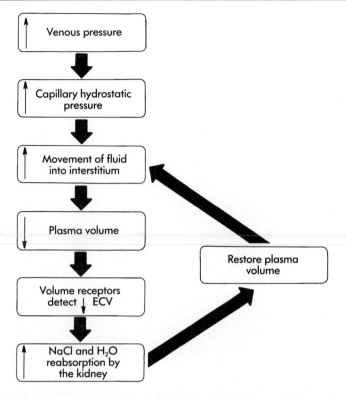

Figure 6-10 ■ Steps involved in the development of edema resulting from an increase in venous pressure (e.g., during heart failure). NaCl and water retention by the kidneys maintains plasma volume allowing the accumulation of fluid in the interstitium. See text for details.

The Role of the Kidneys

In each of the conditions described above, excess fluid accumulates in the interstitium at the expense of the plasma. As a result, if the plasma volume is not maintained near a normal level, this fluid accumulation is self-limiting. Consider the situation that exists with heart failure. Because of decreased cardiac performance, venous pressure is elevated. This raises capillary hydrostatic pressure, and there is net accumulation of fluid in the interstitium. Because the source of this fluid is plasma, and assuming plasma volume is not maintained by some mechanism (see below), plasma volume would decrease. This is turn would decrease venous pressure and capillary hydrostatic pressure, and

movement of fluid into the interstitium would cease.

Figure 6-10 illustrates what occurs when an alteration in the capillary Starling forces causes fluid accumulation in the interstitium. As fluid moves from plasma into the interstitium, plasma volume is decreased. The volume receptors sense this as a decrease in ECV. Appropriate signals are sent to the kidney, resulting in a decrease in the excretion of NaCl and water, and plasma volume is restored. With restoration of plasma volume, and assuming the condition altering the Starling forces still exists (e.g., untreated heart failure), additional fluid will move into the interstitium, and edema will form. This cycle will continue until a new steady state is reached at the capillary level, such that the amount of fluid moving out of the capillary lumen into the interstitium is again balanced by the amount moving in the opposite direction. This steady state can be attained even when the underlying cause is uncorrected. As edema fluid accumulates in the interstitial compartment, the hydrostatic pressure in this compartment increases. This pressure increase occurs as a result of the limited compliance of the surrounding tissue (e.g., skin).* Eventually, the hydrostatic pressure will rise to a level at which net accumulation in the interstitial compartment ceases.

The importance of NaCl retention by the kidneys in edema formation provides two approaches for treatment. The first involves dietary manipulation. The ultimate source of NaCl is the diet. Thus, if dietary intake of NaCl is restricted, the amount that the kidneys can retain is reduced, and edema formation is limited. The second approach is to inhibit the kidneys' ability to retain NaCl. This is accomplished by the use of diuretics, which, as described in Chapter 10, inhibit Na^+ transport mechanisms in the nephron. Thus, Na^+ excretion is increased, and ECF volume is reduced.

■ KEY WORDS AND CONCEPTS

- Effective circulating volume (ECV)
- Natriuresis
- ECV sensors
- Baroreceptors
- Renal sympathetic nerves
- Atrial natriuretic peptide
- Juxtaglomerular apparatus
- Renin-angiotensin-aldosterone system

---

*The situation is analogous to the pressure increase that occurs as a balloon is inflated. Initially, the volume of the balloon increases without a large increase in pressure. However, as the balloon reaches its limit or distensibility, the pressure increases.

- Angiotensinogen
- Converting enzyme
- Aldosterone-induced proteins
- Vasopressin (ADH)
- Euvolemia
- Positive and negative Na^+ balance
- Glomerulotubular balance (GT-balance)
- Starling forces
- Expansion of ECV
- Contraction of ECV
- Edema

■ SELF-STUDY PROBLEMS

1. An individual develops an acute episode of vomiting and diarrhea, and loses 3 kg in body weight over a 24-hour period. A blood sample shows that plasma $[Na^+]$ is normal at 145 mEq/L. Indicate whether the following parameters would be increased, decreased, or unchanged from their values prior to this illness.

Plasma osmolality	_____
ECV	_____
Plasma ADH levels	_____
Urine osmolality	_____
Sensation of thirst	_____

2. An individual is euvolemic and ingests a diet that contains 200 mEq/day of Na^+ on average. What would the Na^+ excretion rate of this individual be over a 24-hour period?

3. Indicate on the following table whether the signals listed are increased or decreased by the indicated change in ECV.

Regulatory factors	Increased ECV	Decreased ECV
Renal sympathetic nerves	_____	_____
ANP	_____	_____
Renin-angiotensin	_____	_____
Aldosterone	_____	_____
Vasopressin	_____	_____

4. A patient with heart failure has developed edema with swelling of the ankles and fluid in the lungs. During the past 2 weeks, the individual's weight has increased by 4 kg. Assuming that the entire weight gain is a result of the accumulation of fluid, calculate the following:

Volume of accumulated fluid: _____ L
Amount of Na⁺ retained by
    the kidneys   _____ mEq

5. As illustrated below, administration of high doses of aldosterone to a normal individual leads to the transient retention of Na^+ by the kidneys. However, after several days, Na^+ excretion increases to its level prior to hormone administration. When the hormone is stopped, Na^+ excretion transiently increases, but returns to its initial level over several days. Delineate the mechanisms involved in these transient changes in Na^+ excretion.

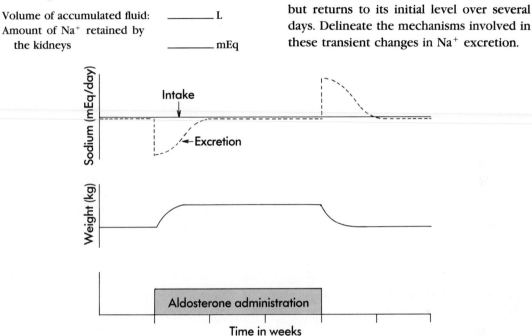

7 Regulation of Potassium Balance

■ **OBJECTIVES**

1. Explain how the body maintains K⁺ homeostasis.
2. Describe the distribution of K⁺ within the body compartments.
3. Identify the hormones and factors that regulate plasma K⁺ levels.
4. Describe the transport pattern of K⁺ along the nephron.
5. Describe the cellular mechanism of K⁺ secretion by the distal tubule and collecting duct, and how secretion is regulated.
6. Explain how plasma K⁺ levels, aldosterone, ADH, tubular fluid flow rate, acid-base balance, and Na⁺ concentration in tubular fluid influence K⁺ secretion.

Potassium, one of the most abundant cations in the body, is critical for many cell functions. Its concentration in cells and extracellular fluid remains constant despite wide fluctuations in dietary K⁺ intake. Two sets of regulatory mechanisms safeguard K⁺ homeostasis: First, several mechanisms regulate internal K⁺ balance, which controls [K⁺] in the intracellular and extracellular fluid. Second, another set of mechanisms holds external K⁺ balance constant by adjusting K⁺ excretion by the kidneys to match dietary K⁺ intake. It is the kidneys that maintain external K⁺ balance. This chapter focuses on the hormones and factors influencing [K⁺] in the intracellular and extracellular fluid compartments *(internal K⁺ balance)* and the hormones and factors regulating the amount of K⁺ in the body *(external K⁺ balance)*.

■ OVERVIEW OF K⁺ HOMEOSTASIS

Total body K⁺ has been estimated at 50 mEq/kg of body weight, or 3,500 mEq for a 70-kg individual. Ninety-eight percent of the K⁺ in the body is located within cells, where its average concentration is 150 mEq/L. A high intracellular [K⁺] is required for many cell functions, including growth and division, enzyme function, acid-base balance, volume regulation, excitability, and contraction (see box on page 111). Only 2% of total body K⁺ is located in the extracellular fluid, where its normal concentration is 4 mEq/L. The large concentration difference across cell membranes (146 mEq/L) is maintained by the operation of Na⁺-K⁺-ATPase. This gradient is important for maintaining the potential difference across cell membranes. Thus, K⁺ is critical for the excitability of nerve

110

and muscle cells, as well as the contractility of cardiac, skeletal, and smooth muscle cells.

When the [K⁺] in the extracellular fluid exceeds 5.5 mEq/L, an individual is *hyperkalemic.* Hyperkalemia reduces the resting membrane potential (the voltage becomes less negative) and increases the excitability of neurons, cardiac cells, and muscle cells (Figure 7-1). Severe, rapid increases in plasma [K⁺] can lead to cardiac arrest and death.

In contrast, when the [K⁺] of the extracellular fluid is less than 3.5 mEq/L, an individual is *hy-* *pokalemic.* A decline in extracellular [K⁺] hyperpolarizes the resting cell membrane potential (the voltage becomes more negative) and reduces the excitability of neurons, cardiac cells, and muscle cells (Figure 7-1). Severe hypokalemia can lead to paralysis, cardiac arrhythmias, decreased ability to concentrate the urine, metabolic alkalosis, increased production of NH_4^+ by the kidneys, and death.

The importance of K⁺ balance is evident in the clinical setting when cardiac arrhythmias are produced by hypokalemia and hyperkalemia. Figure 7-2 shows several electrocardiograms (ECGs) of patients with various levels of [K⁺]. The first sign of hyperkalemia is the appearance of tall, thin T waves. Further increases in [K⁺] prolong the PR interval, depress the ST segment, and lengthen the QRS interval. Finally, as [K⁺] approaches 10 mEq/L, the P wave disappears, the QRS interval broadens, the ECG appears as a sine wave, and the ventricles fi-

---

K⁺ and cell functions

- Growth and division
- Chemical reactions (enzymes)
- Acid-base balance
- Volume regulation
- Excitability and contractility

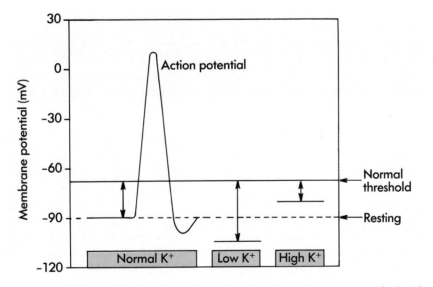

Figure 7-1 ■ The effects of variations in plasma [K⁺] on the resting membrane potential of skeletal muscle. Hyperkalemia causes the membrane potential to approach the threshold potential thereby increasing excitability. Hypokalemia causes the membrane potential to move away from the threshold potential, thereby reducing excitability. Length of double headed arrows indicates the magnitude of difference between resting membrane potential and normal threshold potential.

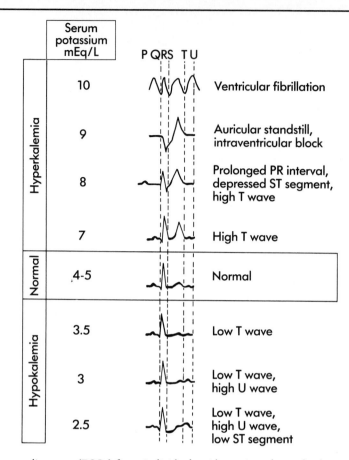

Figure 7-2 ■ Electrocardiograms (ECGs) from individuals with varying plasma [K⁺]. Hyperkalemia increases the height of the T wave and hypokalemia inverts the T wave. See the text for details. (Modified from Barker L, Burton J, and Zieve P: Principles of ambulatory medicine, ed 3, Baltimore, 1991, Williams & Wilkins.)

brillate (i.e., rapid contractions of muscle fibers, but not of the entire ventricle). Hypokalemia prolongs the QT interval, inverts the T wave, and lowers the ST segment. The ECG is a fast, simple way to determine whether changes in plasma [K⁺] influence the heart and other excitable cells. In contrast, plasma [K⁺] measurements by a clinical laboratory require a blood sample, and values are often not immediately available.

K⁺ homeostasis requires that the [K⁺] in the intracellular and extracellular fluid be constant (i.e., internal K⁺ balance) and the total amount of K⁺ in the body be constant (i.e., external K⁺ balance). The factors and hormones maintaining K⁺ homeostasis are reviewed next.

■ INTERNAL K⁺ DISTRIBUTION

After a meal, the K⁺ absorbed by the gastrointestinal tract rapidly enters the extracellular fluid. If all of the K⁺ ingested during a normal meal (~50 mEq) were to remain in the extracellular fluid compartment, plasma [K⁺] would increase by a potentially lethal 3.6 mEq/L (50 mEq of K⁺ added to 14 L of extracellular fluid). This rise in plasma [K⁺] is attenuated by the

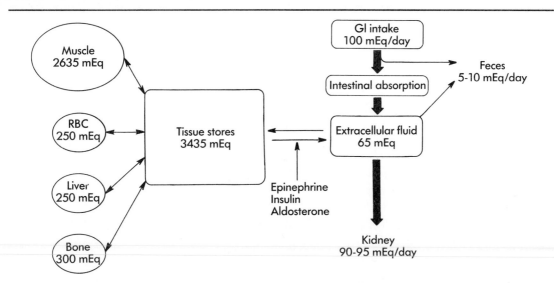

Figure 7-3 ■ Overview of potassium homeostasis. The distribution of K⁺ between the intracellular fluid and the extracellular fluid is regulated by epinephrine, insulin, and aldosterone. These hormones stimulate K⁺ uptake by muscle, red blood cells, liver, and bone, and are secreted when the [K⁺] of the extracellular fluid rises. The amount of K⁺ in the body is regulated by the kidneys. An individual is in balance when the amount absorbed by the gastrointestinal tract and urinary output are equal. The excretion of K⁺ by the kidneys is regulated by several hormones and factors described in the text. Absorption by the gastrointestinal tract is relatively constant. Some K⁺ entering the gastrointestinal tract escapes absorption and some of the absorbed K⁺ is secreted from the extracellular fluid into the lumen of the intestine.

rapid (minutes) uptake of K⁺ into cells. Because K⁺ excretion by the kidneys after a meal is relatively slow (hours), its uptake by cells is essential to prevent life-threatening hyperkalemia. To maintain external K⁺ balance, all of the K⁺ absorbed by the gastrointestinal tract must eventually be excreted by the kidneys. This K⁺ is slowly excreted by the kidneys and, after 6 hours, it is eliminated from the body, thereby maintaining external K⁺ homeostasis.

Several hormones promote the uptake of K⁺ into cells following a rise in plasma [K⁺], thereby preventing dangerous hyperkalemia. As illustrated in Figure 7-3 and the box at right, these hormones include *epinephrine, insulin,* and *aldosterone.* They increase K⁺ uptake into skeletal muscle, liver, bone, and red blood cells by stimulating Na⁺-K⁺-ATPase. Hyperkalemia, subsequent to K⁺ absorption by the gastrointestinal tract, stimulates insulin secretion from

---

Factors influencing the distribution of K⁺ between the intracellular and extracellular fluid

Physiologic: Keep Plasma [K⁺] Constant

Epinephrine
Insulin
Aldosterone

Pathophysiologic: Displace Plasma [K⁺] from Normal

Acid-base balance
Plasma osmolality
Cell lysis
Exercise

---

the pancreas, aldosterone release from the adrenal cortex, and epinephrine secretion from the adrenal medulla. In contrast, hypokalemia inhibits release of these hormones.

Epinephrine

Catecholamines affect the distribution of K^+ across cell membranes by activating α and β_2-adrenergic receptors. Stimulation of α receptors increases plasma $[K^+]$, while stimulation of β_2 receptors decreases it. The importance of β_2 receptors is illustrated by three observations: First, the rise in plasma $[K^+]$ after a K^+-rich meal is greater if the subject has been pretreated with propranolol, a β-adrenergic blocker. Second, the release of epinephrine during stress (e.g., coronary ischemia) can rapidly lower plasma $[K^+]$. Thrid, α receptor activation post-exercise is important for preventing hypokalemia.

Insulin

Insulin also stimulates K^+ uptake into cells. The importance of insulin is illustrated by two observations: first, the rise in plasma $[K^+]$ after a K^+-rich meal is greater in patients with diabetes mellitus (i.e., insulin deficiency). Second, infusion of glucose (to increase insulin levels) or insulin is a form of acute therapy to treat hyperkalemia. Insulin is the most important hormone for causing K^+ uptake into cells following ingestion of K^+ in a meal.

Aldosterone

Aldosterone, like catecholamines and insulin, promotes K^+ uptake into cells. A rise in aldosterone levels (e.g., primary aldosteronism) causes hypokalemia, and a fall in aldosterone levels (e.g., Addison's disease) causes hyperkalemia.

Thus far, the discussion has focused on hormones that regulate the distribution of K^+ across cell membranes. There are other factors that influence K^+ movements across cell membranes; however, they are not homeostatic mechanisms, because they displace plasma $[K^+]$ from normal levels. These factors are summarized in the box on page 113 and are discussed next.

Acid-Base Balance

Changes in acid-base balance significantly affect plasma $[K^+]$. Metabolic acidosis generally increases plasma $[K^+]$, and metabolic alkalosis decreases it, whereas respiratory acid-base disorders do not have appreciable effects on plasma $[K^+]$. For example, metabolic acidosis produced by the addition of inorganic acids (e.g., HCl and H_2SO_4), but not organic acids (e.g., lactic acid and acetic acid), to the extracellular fluid causes an increase of plasma $[K^+]$. Plasma $[K^+]$ increases 0.2 to 1.7 mEq/L for every 0.1 unit fall in pH. The reduced pH promotes movement of H^+ into cells and the reciprocal movement of K^+ out of cells. Metabolic alkalosis has the opposite effect: plasma $[K^+]$ decreases as K^+ moves into cells and H^+ leaves cells. The mechanism responsible for this shift is not fully understood. It has been proposed that the movement of H^+ occurs as the cells buffer changes in the $[H^+]$ of the extracellular fluid (Chapter 8). As H^+ moves across the cell membrane, K^+ moves in the opposite direction; thus, there is no gain or loss of cations across the cell membranes.*

Plasma Osmolality

Plasma osmolality also influences the distribution of K^+ across cell membranes. An increase in the osmolality of the extracellular fluid enhances K^+ release by cells and thus increases extracellular $[K^+]$. The plasma K^+ level may increase by 0.4 to 0.8 mEq/L for a 10 mOsm/kg H_2O elevation in plasma osmolality. Hyposmolality has the opposite action.

---

*Although organic acids produce metabolic acidosis, they do not cause hyperkalemia. Two explanations have been suggested for the inability of organic acids to cause hyperkalemia: First, the organic anion may enter the cell with H^+, thereby eliminating K^+ for H^+ exchange across the membrane. Second, organic anions may stimulate insulin secretion, which drives K^+ into cells, counteracting the direct effect of the acidosis, which moves K^+ out of cells.

As plasma osmolality increases, water will leave cells due to the osmotic gradient across the plasma membrane. Water continues to leave cells until the intracellular osmolality becomes equal to that in the plasma. Loss of water causes cells to shrink, and cell $[K^+]$ to rise, which provides a driving force for K^+ efflux from the cells. This sequence results in a rise in plasma $[K^+]$. A fall in plasma osmolality has the opposite effect.

Cell Lysis

Cell lysis causes hyperkalemia. Severe trauma (e.g., burns) and some diseases, such as tumor lysis syndrome and rhabdomyolysis (i.e., destruction of skeletal muscle), cause cell destruction and the release of K^+ (and other cell solutes) into the extracellular fluid. In addition, gastric ulcers cause seepage of red blood cells into the gastrointestinal tract. These cells are digested, and the K^+ released from them is absorbed, causing hyperkalemia.

Exercise

K^+ is released from skeletal muscle cells during exercise; the amount released and the ensuing hyperkalemia depend on the degree of exercise. Plasma $[K^+]$ increases by 0.3 mEq/L with slow walking and may increase by up to 2 mEq/L with strenuous exercise. These changes in plasma $[K^+]$ usually produce no symptoms and are reversed after several minutes of rest. However, for individuals with disorders in internal K^+ balance (certain endocrine disorders), impaired ability to excrete K^+ (renal failure), or those on certain medications, exercise can lead to potentially life-threatening hyperkalemia. For example, individuals taking β-adrenergic blockers for hypertension can raise plasma $[K^+]$ by 2 to 4 mEq/L during exercise.

It is important to recognize that acid-base balance, plasma osmolality, cell lysis, and exercise do not maintain plasma $[K^+]$ at a normal value and therefore do not contribute to K^+ homeostasis. The extent to which these pathophysiological states alter plasma $[K^+]$ depends on the integrity of the homeostatic mechanisms regulating plasma $[K^+]$ (e.g., secretion of epinephrine, insulin, and aldosterone).

■ EXTERNAL K^+ BALANCE: EXCRETION OF K^+ BY THE KIDNEYS

The kidneys play the major role in maintaining external body K^+ balance. As illustrated in Figure 7-3, they excrete 92% of the K^+ ingested in the diet. Excretion is equivalent to intake even when intake increases by as much as 20 times. This equivalence between urinary excretion and dietary intake underscores the importance of the kidneys in maintaining K^+ homeostasis. Although small amounts of K^+ are lost each day in the feces and perspiration (~8% of the K^+ ingested in the diet), this amount is essentially constant and is not regulated; therefore, it is much less important than K^+ excretion by the kidneys.* *The primary event is determining urinary K^+ excretion is K^+ secretion from the blood into the tubular fluid by the cells of the distal tubule and collecting duct system.* The transport pattern of K^+ by the major nephron segments is illustrated in Figure 7-4.

Because K^+ is not bound to plasma proteins, it is freely filtered by the glomerulus. Normally, urinary K^+ excretion is 15% of the amount filtered. Accordingly, K^+ is reabsorbed along the nephron under normal conditions. When dietary K^+ intake is augmented, however, K^+ excretion can exceed the amount filtered, indicating that K^+ is also secreted.

The proximal tubule reabsorbs 67% of the filtered K^+, Henle's loop reabsorbs 20%. In both

---

*With diarrhea, K^+ loss in the feces increases and becomes an important route for K^+ loss from the body.

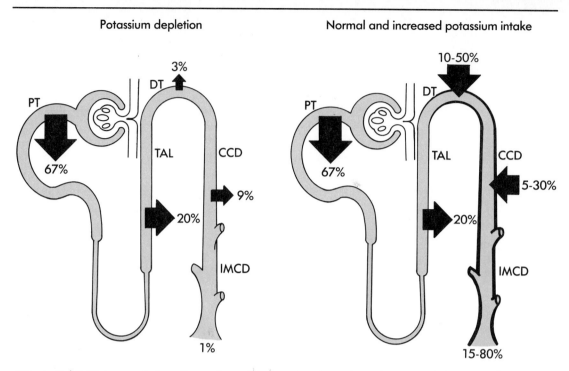

Figure 7-4 ■ K$^+$ transport along the nephron. K$^+$ excretion depends on the rate and direction of K$^+$ secretion by the distal tubule and the collecting duct. Percentages refer to the amount of filtered K$^+$ reabsorbed or secreted by each nephron segment. **Left,** Dietary K$^+$ depletion. An amount of K$^+$ equal to 1% of the filtered load of K$^+$ is excreted. **Right,** Normal and increased dietary K$^+$ intake. An amount of K$^+$ equal to 15% to 80% of the filtered load is excreted. *PT,* proximal tubule; *TAL,* thick ascending limb; DT, distal tubule; *CCD,* collecting duct; *IMCD,* inner medullary collecting duct.

segments, reabsorption is a constant fraction of the amount filtered. In contrast to these segments, which are capable of only reabsorbing K$^+$, the distal tubule and collecting duct have the dual capacity to reabsorb and secrete K$^+$. The rate of K$^+$ reabsorption or secretion by these segments is variable and depends on several hormones and other factors. When K$^+$ intake is normal (100 mEq/day), it is secreted by these segments. A rise in dietary K$^+$ intake increases K$^+$ secretion, such that the amount of K$^+$ appearing in the urine can reach an amount equivalent to 80% of that filtered (Figure 7-4). In contrast, a low K$^+$ diet activates K$^+$ reabsorption along the distal tubule and collecting

duct, such that urinary excretion falls to 1% of the K$^+$ filtered by the glomerulus (Figure 7-4). The kidneys are not able to reduce K$^+$ excretion to the same low levels as those seen for Na$^+$. Therefore, hypokalemia can develop in individuals on K$^+$-deficient diets.

Because the magnitude and direction of K$^+$ transport by the distal tubule and collecting duct are variable, the overall rate of urinary K$^+$ excretion is determined by these tubular segments. The remainder of this section focuses on the mechanisms of K$^+$ transport by the distal tubule and collecting duct, and the factors and hormones that regulate K$^+$ transport by these segments.

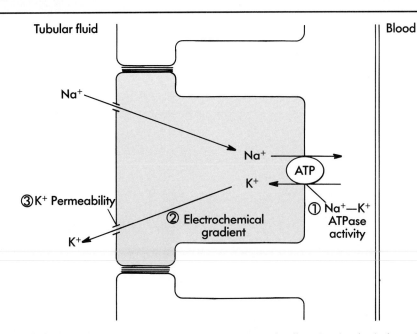

Tubular fluid | Blood

Na⁺

Na⁺

ATP

K⁺

③ K⁺ Permeability

② Electrochemical gradient

① Na⁺—K⁺ ATPase activity

K⁺

Figure 7-5 ■ Cellular mechanism of K⁺ secretion by the principal cell in the distal tubule and collecting duct. The numbers indicate the sites where K⁺ secretion is regulated. *1*, Na⁺-K⁺-ATPase; *2*, Electrochemical gradient (driving force) for K⁺ efflux across the apical membrane; and *3*, The K⁺ permeability of the apical membrane.

■ CELLULAR MECHANISMS OF K⁺ TRANSPORT BY THE DISTAL TUBULE AND COLLECTING DUCT

Figure 7-5 shows the cellular mechanism of K⁺ secretion by principal cells in the distal tubule and collecting duct. Secretion from blood into tubular fluid is a two-step process involving uptake across the basolateral membrane via Na⁺-K⁺-ATPase and diffusion of K⁺ from the cell into the tubular fluid. Na⁺-K⁺-ATPase creates a high intracellular [K⁺], which provides the chemical force for K⁺ exit across the apical membrane through K⁺ channels. Although these channels are also present in the basolateral membrane, K⁺ preferentially leaves the cell across the apical membrane and enters the tubular fluid. There are two reasons for this: first, the electrochemical gradient of K⁺ across the apical membrane favors the downhill movement into the tubular fluid. Second, the perme-

ability of the apical membrane to K⁺ is greater than that of the basolateral membrane.

As illustrated in Figure 7-5, the three major parameters controlling the rate of K⁺ secretion by the distal tubule and collecting duct are:
1. The activity of Na⁺-K⁺-ATPase.
2. The electrochemical gradient (driving force) for K⁺ efflux across the apical membrane.
3. The permeability of the apical membrane to K⁺.

Every change in K⁺ secretion results from an alteration in one or more of these parameters.

In contrast, the cellular pathways and mechanisms of K⁺ reabsorption in the distal tubule and collecting duct are not fully understood. Evidence suggests that K⁺ is reabsorbed by intercalated cells via an H⁺-K⁺-ATPase located in the apical membrane. This transporter mediates K⁺ uptake across the apical membrane, but the

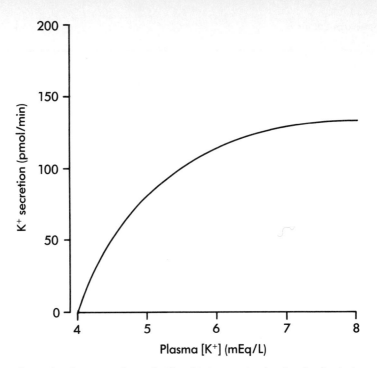

Figure 7-6 ■ The relationship between plasma [K⁺] and K⁺ secretion by the distal tubule and the cortical collecting duct.

pathway of K⁺ exit from intercalated cells into the blood is unknown. Reabsorption of K⁺ is activated by a low K⁺ diet.

■ REGULATION OF K⁺ EXCRETION

Regulation of K⁺ excretion occurs primarily as a result of alterations in K⁺ secretion by the principal cells of the distal tubule and collecting duct. The box lists the major factors and hormones that modulate K⁺ secretion by these cells. Plasma [K⁺] and aldosterone are the major physiological regulators of K⁺ secretion. ADH, the flow rate of tubular fluid, acid-base balance, and tubular fluid [Na⁺] also modify K⁺ secretion; however, they are less important than plasma [K⁺] and aldosterone.

Plasma [K⁺]

Plasma [K⁺] is an important determinant of K⁺ secretion by the distal tubule and collecting duct. Figure 7-6 diagrams the relationship between plasma [K⁺] and K⁺ secretion by the distal tubule. Hyperkalemia (e.g., high K⁺

> ## *Major factors and hormones regulating K⁺ secretion by the distal tubule and collecting duct*
>
> - Plasma [K⁺]
> - Aldosterone
> - Flow rate of tubular fluid
> - Antidiuretic hormone
> - Acid-base balance
> - [Na⁺] of tubular fluid

diet or rhabdomyolysis) stimulates secretion in minutes. Several mechanisms are involved: First, hyperkalemia stimulates Na⁺-K⁺-ATPase, thereby increasing K⁺ uptake across the basolateral membrane. This raises intracellular [K⁺], which increases the driving force for K⁺ exit across the apical membrane. Second, hyperkalemia increases the permeability of the apical membrane to K⁺. Third, hyperkalemia stimu-

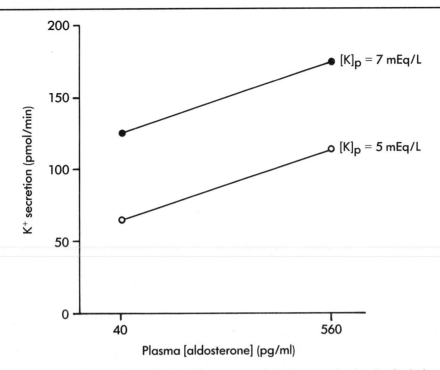

Figure 7-7 ■ The relationship between plasma aldosterone and K$^+$ secretion by the distal tubule and the cortical collecting duct. Note that the effects of plasma [K$^+$] and aldosterone on K$^+$ secretion are additive.

lates aldosterone secretion by the adrenal cortex, which acts synergistically with K$^+$ to stimulate K$^+$ secretion.

Hypokalemia (e.g., low K$^+$ diet or diarrhea), decreases K$^+$ secretion by actions opposite those described for hyperkalemia. Hypokalemia inhibits Na$^+$-K$^+$-ATPase, decreases the driving force for K$^+$ efflux across the apical membrane, reduces the permeability of the apical membrane to K$^+$, and causes a reduction in plasma [aldosterone].

Aldosterone

Figure 7-7 illustrates the effect of aldosterone on K$^+$ secretion by the distal tubule and collecting duct. In addition to stimulating Na$^+$ reabsorption, aldosterone enhances K$^+$ secretion by increasing the amount of Na$^+$-K$^+$-AT-Pase in principal cells, thus elevating cell [K$^+$].

Aldosterone also increases the driving force for K$^+$ exit across the apical membrane and increases the permeability of the apical membrane to K$^+$. Aldosterone secretion is increased by hyperkalemia and angiotensin II (following activation of the renin-angiotensin system), and decreased by hypokalemia and ANP. Stimulation of K$^+$ secretion by aldosterone occurs after a one-hour lag period, and it attains its highest level after one day.

Flow Rate of Tubular Fluid

As shown in Figure 7-8, a rise in the flow rate of tubular fluid (e.g., diuretic treatment or extracellular fluid volume expansion) rapidly stimulates K$^+$ secretion. Conversely, a fall in the flow rate (e.g., extracellular fluid volume contraction) reduces secretion. Increases in flow rate are more effective in stimulating K$^+$ secretion

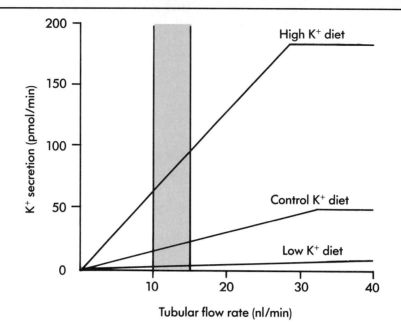

Figure 7-8 ■ Relationship between tubular flow rate and K⁺ secretion by the distal tubule and cortical collecting duct. A high K⁺ diet increases the slope of the relationship between flow rate and secretion and increases the maximum rate of secretion. A low K⁺ diet has the opposite effects. Shaded bar indicates the flow rate under most physiological conditions.

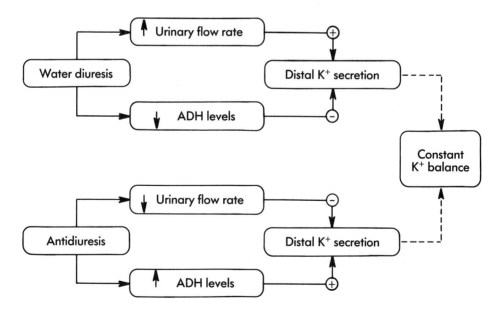

Figure 7-9 ■ Dual effects of ADH on K⁺ secretion by the distal tubule and cortical collecting duct. Because the two effects oppose each other, net K⁺ secretion is not affected by ADH.

as dietary K$^+$ intake is increased from a low to high K$^+$ diet (Figure 7-8). Alterations in the flow rate influence K$^+$ secretion by changing the driving force of potassium exit across the apical membrane. As potassium is secreted into the tubular fluid, the [K$^+$] of the fluid increases. This decreases the driving force for K$^+$ exit across the apical membrane, thereby reducing the rate of secretion. An increase in flow rate minimizes the rise in tubular fluid [K$^+$] as the secreted K$^+$ is washed downstream. As a result, K$^+$ secretion is stimulated by an increase in the flow rate of tubular fluid. Because diuretic drugs increase the flow rate through the distal tubule and collecting duct, they enhance urinary K$^+$ excretion (see Chapter 10). In contrast, a decline in flow rate inhibits K$^+$ secretion by facilitating the rise in tubular fluid [K$^+$].

Antidiuretic Hormone

ADH increases the driving force for K$^+$ exit across the apical membrane of principal cells in the distal tubule and collecting duct. However, because it also decreases the flow rate of tubular fluid, which reduces K$^+$ secretion, ADH does not change K$^+$ secretion by the distal tubule and collecting duct. As illustrated in Figure 7-9, changes in ADH levels do not alter urinary K$^+$ excretion, because the stimulatory effect of ADH on K$^+$ secretion is offset by the inhibitory effect of decreased tubular flow rate. If ADH did not increase the electrochemical gradient favoring K$^+$ secretion, urinary K$^+$ excretion would fall with increased ADH levels, and K$^+$ balance would be modulated by alterations in water balance.

Acid-Base Balance

Another factor that regulates K$^+$ secretion is the [H$^+$] of the extracellular fluid. Acute alterations (over a period of minutes to hours) in plasma pH influence K$^+$ secretion by the distal tubule and collecting duct. As depicted in Figure 7-10, alkalosis increases secretion, and acidosis decreases secretion. Acidosis reduces K$^+$ secretion by two actions: inhibiting Na$^+$-K$^+$-

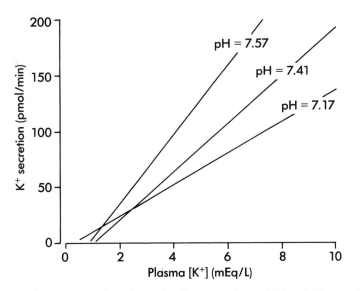

Figure 7-10 ■ Effect of plasma pH on the relationship between plasma [K$^+$] and K$^+$ secretion by the distal tubule and the cortical collecting duct.

2

ATPase, which reduces K^+ uptake into the cell, thereby reducing the driving force for K^+ exit across the apical membrane, and by reducing the permeability of the apical membrane to K^+. Alkalosis has the opposite effects.

The effect of metabolic acidosis on K^+ excretion is time-dependent. When metabolic acidosis is prolonged for several days, urinary K^+ excretion is stimulated. This occurs because chronic metabolic acidosis inhibits water and NaCl reabsorption by the proximal tubule, thereby increasing the flow of tubular fluid through the distal tubule and collecting duct. This rise in flow rate offsets the effects of acidosis on cell $[K^+]$ and apical membrane permeability, such that K^+ secretion rises. Thus, metabolic acidosis can either inhibit or stimulate potassium excretion, depending upon the duration of the disturbance.

$[Na^+]$ of Tubular Fluid

The $[Na^+]$ of tubular fluid can, under some conditions, be an important determinant of K^+ secretion. A rise in $[Na^+]$ stimulates secretion, whereas a fall in its concentration has the opposite effect. An increase in the $[Na^+]$ of tubular fluid enhances Na^+ movement across the apical membrane of principal cells and increases intracellular $[Na^+]$. This stimulates Na^+-K^+-ATPase and accelerates K^+ uptake across the basolateral membrane. The rise in intracellular $[K^+]$ in turn increases the favorable electrochemical gradient for K^+ exit across the apical membrane, thereby enhancing K^+ secretion. The opposite occurs with a decrease in tubular fluid $[Na^+]$.

■ KEY WORDS AND CONCEPTS

- Hyperkalemia
- Hypokalemia
- Internal K^+ balance
- Insulin
- Epinephrine
- Plasma osmolality
- Acid-base balance
- External K^+ balance
- Cellular mechanisms of K^+ secretion by the distal tubule and collecting duct
- Hormones and factors regulating K^+ excretion
- Aldosterone
- ADH
- Plasma $[K^+]$
- Tubular fluid flow rate
- Tubular fluid $[Na^+]$

■ SELF-STUDY PROBLEMS

1. What would happen to the rise in plasma $[K^+]$ following an intravenous K^+ load if the subject had a combination of sympathetic blockade and insulin deficiency?
2. What effect would aldosterone deficiency have on urinary K^+ excretion? What would happen to plasma $[K^+]$, and what effect would this have on K^+ excretion?
3. Describe the homeostatic mechanisms involved in maintaining plasma $[K^+]$ following ingestion of a K^+-rich meal.
4. If both the GFR and filtered load of K^+ declined by 50%, would the kidneys be able to maintain K^+ balance? If so, how would this occur? If not, would the subject become hyperkalemic?

8 Regulation of Acid-Base Balance

■ OBJECTIVES

1. Explain the chemistry of the CO_2/HCO_3^- buffer system and its role as the primary physiological buffer of extracellular fluid.
2. Describe the metabolic processes that produce acid and alkali, and their net effect on systemic acid-base balance. Distinguish between volatile and nonvolatile acids.
3. Explain the concept of net acid excretion by the kidneys, and the importance of urinary buffers in this process.
4. Describe the mechanisms of H^+ secretion in the various segments of the nephron and how these mechanisms are regulated.
5. Distinguish between the reabsorption of filtered HCO_3^- and the formation of new HCO_3^-.
6. Describe the mechanisms of ammonia production and excretion by the kidneys, and explain their importance in renal acid excretion and thus systemic acid-base balance.
7. Describe the three general mechanisms used by the body to defend against acid-base disturbances:
   a. Intracellular and extracellular buffering
   b. Respiratory compensation
   c. Renal compensation
8. Distinguish between simple metabolic and respiratory acid-base disorders, and the body's response to them.
9. Analyze acid-base disorders, and distinguish between simple and mixed disorders.

The concentration of H^+ in the body fluids is low compared to that of other ions. For example, Na^+ is present at a concentration some three million times greater than that of H^+ ($[Na^+] = 140$ mEq/L; $[H^+] = 40$ nEq/L). Because of the low $[H^+]$ of the body fluids, it is commonly expressed as the negative logarithm, or pH. Table 8-1 lists $[H^+]$ and corresponding pH over the physiological range.

Many of the body's metabolic functions are exquisitely sensitive to pH, and normal function can occur only within a very narrow range. The pH range that is generally compatible with life is 6.8 to 7.8 (160 to 16) nEq/L of H^+). This chapter examines the mechanisms the body uses to maintain the pH of the body fluids within this normal range, with special emphasis placed on the role of the kidneys.

■ THE CO_2/HCO_3^- BUFFER SYSTEM

Quantitatively, HCO_3^- is the most important buffer in the extracellular fluid (normal plasma $[HCO_3^-] \cong 24$ mEq/L). The CO_2/HCO_3^- *buffer system* differs from other buffer systems of the

Table 8-1 ■ **Relationship between pH and [H⁺]**

pH	[H⁺], nEq/L
7.8	16
7.7	20
7.6	26
7.5	32
7.4	40
7.3	50
7.2	63
7.1	80
7.0	100
6.9	125
6.8	160

body (e.g., phosphate), because it is under the dual regulation of the lung and kidneys. This can best be understood by considering the reactions of CO_2 in water.

$$CO_2 + H_2O \overset{CA}{\leftrightarrow} H_2CO_3 \leftrightarrow H^+ + HCO_3^- \quad (8\text{-}1)$$

The first reaction (hydration/dehydration of CO_2) is the rate-limiting step. This reaction, which is normally slow, is greatly accelerated in the presence of the enzyme *carbonic anhydrase (CA)*. The second reaction, the ionization of H_2CO_3, is virtually instantaneous.

To quantitate these reactions, it is simpler to consider H^+ and HCO_3^- as products, and CO_2 and H_2CO_3 as reactants. Thus:

$$K' = \frac{[H^+][HCO_3^-]}{[CO_2][H_2CO_3]} \quad (8\text{-}2)$$

Because this simplification combines the dissociation reaction $(H_2CO_3 \leftrightarrow H^+ + HCO_3^-)$ with hydration/dehydration reaction $(CO_2 + H_2O \leftrightarrow H_2CO_3)$, K' is not a true dissociation constant. Instead, it is termed an apparent dissociation constant. The value of K' is dependent upon temperature and solution composition. For plasma at 37° C, K' has a value of $10^{-6.1}$ ($pK' = 6.1$).

The terms in the denominator of Equation 8-

2 represent the total amount of CO_2 dissolved in solution. Most of this CO_2 is in the gas form, with only 0.3% being H_2CO_3. Because the amount of CO_2 in solution depends on its partial pressure (P_{CO_2}) and solubility (α), Equation 8-2 can be rewritten as*:

$$K' = \frac{[H^+][HCO_3^-]}{\alpha P_{CO_2}} \quad (8\text{-}3)$$

For plasma at 37° C, $\alpha = 0.03$.

A more useful form of this equation is obtained by solving for $[H^+]$:

$$[H^+] = \frac{K'\alpha P_{CO_2}}{[HCO_3^-]} \text{ or } [H^+] = 24\,\frac{P_{CO_2}}{[HCO_3^-]} \quad (8\text{-}4)$$

Taking the negative logarithm of both sides of the equation yields:

$$-\log[H^+] = \frac{-\log[K'] + -\log\alpha P_{CO_2}}{-\log[HCO_3^-]} \quad (8\text{-}5)$$

$$pH = pK' + \log\frac{[HCO_3^-]}{\alpha P_{CO_2}} \text{ or} \quad (8\text{-}6)$$

$$pH = 6.1 + \log\frac{[HCO_3^-]}{0.03\,P_{CO_2}}$$

Equation 8-6 is the *Henderson-Hasselbalch equation.* Inspection of it shows that the pH of extracellular fluid (ECF) varies when either $[HCO_3^-]$ or P_{CO_2} is altered. Disturbances of acid-base balance that result from a change in ECF $[HCO_3^-]$ are termed *metabolic acid-base disorders,* whereas those resulting from a change in P_{CO_2} are termed *respiratory acid-base disorders.* These disorders are considered in more detail in a subsequent section. The kidney is primarily responsible for regulating $[HCO_3^-]$, while the lungs control P_{CO_2}.

■ METABOLIC PRODUCTION OF ACID AND ALKALI

In a normal individual, the metabolism of dietary food stuffs produces a number of substances that can impact on acid-base status.

---

*α is not strictly a gas solubility constant; rather, it is a constant that relates the P_{CO_2} to the total concentration of H_2CO_3 and the dissolved CO_2.

When insulin is present and the tissues are adequately perfused, cellular metabolism of carbohydrates and fats produces large quantities of CO_2 (15 to 20 mol/day).* This CO_2, which is a potential acid in the body fluids (as H_2CO_3), is termed *volatile acid,* and is excreted from the body by the lungs. In addition, the normal diet contains a number of constituents whose metabolism produces acids other than CO_2. These are termed *nonvolatile acids.*

Metabolites of amino acids constitute a major portion of nonvolatile acid production. The sulfur-containing amino acids cysteine and methionine yield sulfuric acid when metabolized, whereas hydrochloric acid results from the metabolism of the cationic amino acids lysine, arginine, and histidine. This acid production is partially offset by the metabolism of the anionic amino acids aspartate and glutamate, which results in the production of HCO_3^-. Considering all amino acid metabolism, approximately 100 mmol/day of nonvolatile acid is produced (assuming a 100 g/day intake of protein).

Phosphate (as $H_2PO_4^-$) constitutes another nonvolatile acid load to the body. Typically, the acid load associated with phosphate ingestion is in the range of 30 mmol/day.

Finally, the diet contains a number of organic anions (e.g., citrate) that produce HCO_3^- when metabolized. On average, the metabolism of these anions results in the production of approximately 60 mmol/day of HCO_3^-.

Table 8-2 shows the production of nonvolatile acids and HCO_3^- on a typical diet. On balance, acid production exceeds HCO_3^- production, with the net effect being the addition of approximately 70 mmol/day of nonvolatile acid to the body. Expressed in terms of body weight, nonvolatile acid production equals 1 mmol/day/kg. It should be emphasized that the production of nonvolatile acids is highly depen-

*In the absence of insulin, or when tissue hypoxia exists, carbohydrates and fats are incompletely metabolized. When this occurs, large quantities of nonvolatile acids are produced (e.g., lactic acid and β-hydroxybutyric acid).

Table 8-2 ■ Metabolic production of nonvolatile acid and alkali from the diet

Food source	Acid/alkali produced	Quantity (mEq/day)
Carbohydrates	Normally none	0
Fats	Normally none	0
Amino acids		
a. Sulfur-containing[1]	H_2SO_4	
b. Cationic[2]	HCl	100
c. Anionic[3]	HCO_3^-	
Organic anions	HCO_3^-	−60
Phosphate	$H_2PO_4^-$	30
Total		70

1. Cysteine, methionine
2. Lysine, arginine, histidine
3. Aspartate, glutamate

dent upon the diet. For example, acid production can be less on a vegetarian diet.

The nonvolatile acids produced during metabolism do not circulate as free acids, but are immediately buffered.

$$H_2SO_4 + 2NaHCO_3 \leftrightarrow Na_2SO_4 + 2CO_2 + 2H_2O \quad \textbf{(8-7)}$$

$$HCl + NaHCO_3 \leftrightarrow NaCl + CO_2 + H_2O \quad \textbf{(8-8)}$$

This titration process yields the Na^+ salts of the strong acids and removes HCO_3^- from ECF. *In order to maintain acid-base balance, the kidney must excrete these Na^+ salts and replenish the HCO_3^- lost by titration.*

■ OVERVIEW OF RENAL ACID EXCRETION

To maintain acid-base balance, the kidneys must excrete an amount of acid equal to nonvolatile acid production. In addition, they must prevent the loss of HCO_3^- in the urine. This latter task is quantitatively more important, because the filtered load of HCO_3^- is approximately 4,320 mEq/day (24 mEq/L × 180 L/day = 4,320 mEq/day), compared to only 70 mEq/day of nonvolatile acid excretion.

Both the reabsorption of filtered HCO_3^- and the excretion of acid are accomplished through the process of H^+ secretion by the nephrons. Thus, in a single day the nephrons must secrete approximately 4,390 mEq of H^+ into the tubular fluid. Most of the H^+ does not leave the body in the urine, but serves to reabsorb the filtered load of HCO_3^-. Only 70 mEq is excreted. As a result of this acid excretion, the urine is normally acidic.

Theoretically, the kidneys could excrete nonvolatile acids and replenish the HCO_3^- lost during titration by reversing the reactions shown in Equations 8-7 and 8-8. But, because the pKs of these acids are so low, this process would require a urine pH of 1. However, the minimum urine pH attainable by the kidneys is only 4.0 to 4.5. Consequently, the kidneys cannot excrete the free acids, but must excrete their Na^+ salts while excreting H^+ with other urinary buffers. The two major urinary buffers are *ammonia* (NH_3/NH_4^+) and phosphate ($HPO_4^=/H_2PO_4^-$). The urinary phosphate and, to a lesser degree, other buffer species (e.g, creatinine) are collectively termed *titratable acid.*

The overall process of *net acid excretion (NAE)* by the kidney can be quantitated as follows:

$$NAE = [(U_{NH_4^+} \times \dot{V}) + (U_{TA} \times \dot{V})] - (U_{HCO_3^-} \times \dot{V}) \quad (8\text{-}9)$$

where: $U_{NH_4^+} \times \dot{V}$ and $U_{TA} \times \dot{V}$ are the rates of H^+ excretion (mEq/day) as NH_4^+ and titratable acid (TA); and $U_{HCO_3^-} \times \dot{V}$ is the amount of HCO_3^- lost in the urine (equivalent to adding H^+ to the body). *To maintain acid-base balance, net acid excretion must equal nonvolatile acid production.*

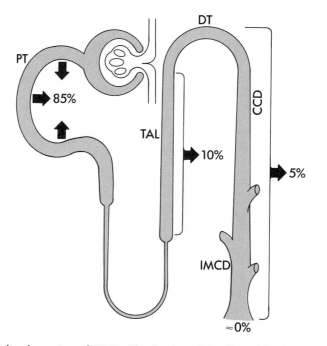

Figure 8-1 ■ Segmental reabsorption of HCO_3^-. The fraction of the filtered load of HCO_3^- reabsorbed by the various segments of the nephron is shown. Normally, the entire filtered load of HCO_3^- is reabsorbed. *PT*, proximal tubule; *TAL*, thick ascending limb; *DT*, distal tubule; *CCD*, cortical collecting duct; *IMCD*, inner medullary collecting duct.

■ HCO₃⁻ REABSORPTION ALONG THE NEPHRON

Figure 8-1 illustrates HCO_3^- reabsorption along the length of the nephron. Because this process prevents HCO_3^- loss in the urine, it is frequently referred to as *reabsorption of filtered HCO_3^-*.

Approximately 85% of the filtered load of HCO_3^- is reabsorbed in the proximal tubule. The cellular mechanisms involved in reabsorption are illustrated in Figure 8-2. The apical membrane of the proximal tubule cell contains an Na^+-H^+ antiporter that secretes H^+ into the tubular fluid using the energy in the lumen-to-cell Na^+ gradient. Recent evidence indicates that a portion of H^+ secretion is also mediated by an H^+-ATPase. Within the cell, H^+ and HCO_3^- are produced in a reaction catalyzed by carbonic anhydrase (see Equation 8-1). The H^+ is secreted into the tubular fluid, whereas the HCO_3^- exits the cell across the basolateral membrane

and returns to the peritubular blood.

HCO_3^- does not simply diffuse from the cell across the basolateral membrane; instead, its movement is coupled to other ions. The majority of HCO_3^- exits via a symporter that couples the efflux of 3 Na^+ with each HCO_3^-. Additionally, some of the HCO_3^- exits in exchange for Cl^- (Cl^--HCO_3^- antiporter). Within the tubular fluid, the secreted H^+ combines with the filtered HCO_3^- to form H_2CO_3. This is rapidly converted to CO_2 and H_2O by carbonic anhydrase present in the apical membrane and exposed to the tubular fluid contents. Because the tubule is highly permeable to CO_2 and H_2O, they are rapidly reabsorbed. The net effect of this process is that, for each HCO_3^- removed from the tubular fluid, one HCO_3^- appears in the peritubular blood.

An additional 10% of the filtered load of HCO_3^- is reabsorbed by Henle's loop. The majority of this HCO_3^- is reabsorbed by the cells of the thick ascending limb. The mechanism for

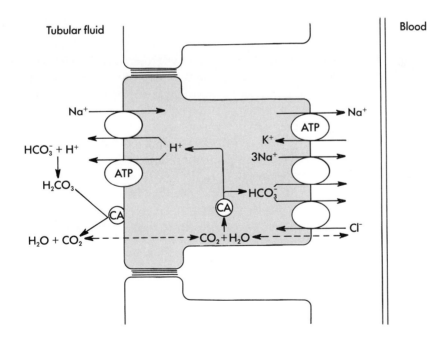

Figure 8-2 ■ Cellular mechanism for reabsorption of filtered HCO_3^- by cells of the proximal tubule. *CA*, carbonic anhydrase.

Tubular fluid

Blood

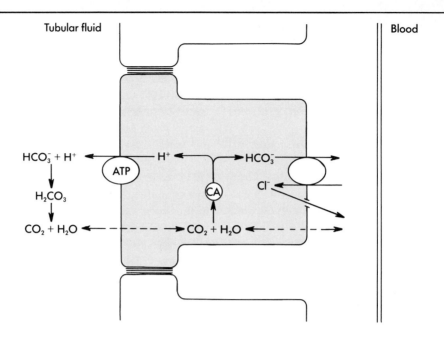

Figure 8-3 ■ Cellular mechanism for reabsorption of filtered HCO_3^- by the intercalated cell of the collecting duct. *CA*, carbonic anhydrase.

HCO_3^- reabsorption by the thick ascending limb cells appears to be similar to that described for the proximal tubule. H^+ is secreted into the tubular fluid by an apical membrane Na^+-H^+ antiporter. HCO_3^- exits the cell across the basolateral membrane coupled to Na^+ ($3Na^+$-$1HCO_3^-$ symporter) and returns to the peritubular blood.

The distal tubule and collecting duct reabsorb the small amount of HCO_3^- that escapes reabsorption by the proximal tubule and Henle's loop (5% of the filtered load). The mechanism by which this occurs does not depend upon Na^+ (i.e., apical membrane Na^+-H^+ antiporter), as is the case in the earlier nephron segments. Figure 8-3 shows the mechanism of HCO_3^- reabsorption by the collecting duct. Here, H^+ secretion occurs via the intercalated cell (see Chapter 2). Within that cell, H^+ and HCO_3^- are produced by the hydration of CO_2; a reaction that is catalyzed by carbonic anhydrase. The H^+ is se-

creted into the tubular fluid by an apical membrane H^+-ATPase. The HCO_3^- exits the cell across the basolateral membrane in exchange for Cl^- (Cl^--HCO_3^- antiporter) and enters the peritubular capillary blood. The apical membrane of the collecting duct cells has a low permeability to H^+, and the pH of the tubular fluid can be rendered quite acidic. Indeed, the most acidic tubular fluid along the nephron (pH = 4.0 to 4.5) is produced here. By comparison, the permeability of the proximal tubule to H^+ and HCO_3^- is much higher, and the tubular fluid pH falls to only 6.5 in this segment.

■ REGULATION OF HCO_3^- REABSORPTION

HCO_3^- reabsorption is regulated by several factors (Table 8-3), which act at both the proximal tubule and collecting duct.

Because of glomerulotubular balance, any change in the filtered load of HCO_3^-, as a result of alterations in GFR, is matched by an appropriate change in HCO_3^- reabsorption by the proximal tubule. Thus, proximal tubule HCO_3^- reabsorption increases with an increase in filtered load and decreases when the filtered load is reduced.

Table 8-3 ■ **Factors regulating H⁺ secretion (HCO_3^- reabsorption) by the nephron**

Factor	Nephron site of action
Increasing H⁺ Secretion	
Increase in filtered load of HCO_3^-	Proximal tubule
Decrease in ECF volume	Proximal tubule
Decrease in plasma $[HCO_3^-]$ (↓ pH)	Proximal tubule, thick ascending limb of Henle's loop, and collecting duct
Increase in blood P_{CO_2}	Proximal tubule, thick ascending limb of Henle's loop, and collecting duct
Aldosterone	Collecting duct
Decreasing H⁺ secretion	
Decrease in filtered load of HCO_3^-	Proximal tubule
Increase in ECF volume	Proximal tubule
Increase in plasma $[HCO_3^-]$ (↑ pH)	Proximal tubule, thick ascending limb of Henle's loop, and collecting duct
Decrease in blood P_{CO_2}	Proximal tubule, thick ascending limb of Henle's loop, and collecting duct

The major fraction of proximal tubule HCO_3^- reabsorption occurs by the Na^+-H^+ antiporter located in the apical membrane of the cells. Consequently, factors that regulate Na^+ homeostasis (see Chapter 6) alter HCO_3^- reabsorption secondarily. Thus, expansion of ECF, which inhibits proximal tubule Na^+ reabsorption, also decreases the reabsorption of HCO_3^-. Conversely, HCO_3^- reabsorption is enhanced when ECF is decreased.

As might be expected, changes in systemic acid-base balance also affect HCO_3^- reabsorption. Systemic acidosis, whether produced by a decrease in plasma $[HCO_3^-]$ (metabolic) or an increase in the P_{CO_2} (respiratory), stimulates HCO_3^- reabsorption in the proximal tubule, Henle's loop, and the collecting duct. This stimulation is believed to occur as a result of acidification of the intracellular fluid, which in turn produces a more favorable cell-to-lumen H^+ gradient and enhances H^+ secretion. There is also evidence, at least in the collecting duct, that acidification of the intracellular fluid results in the insertion of more H^+-ATPase into the apical membrane of the intercalated cells. With more H^+-ATPase, H^+ secretion and thus HCO_3^- reabsorption are enhanced. Conversely, metabolic and respiratory alkalosis inhibit HCO_3^- reabsorption in the proximal tubule, Henle's loop, and the collecting duct. The mechanisms involved are thought to be the opposite of those for stimulation of HCO_3^- reabsorption with acidosis.

Aldosterone is a major regulatory factor for HCO_3^- reabsorption. Aldosterone stimulates H^+ secretion by the intercalated cells of the collecting duct. This reflects both the direct action of the hormone on the intercalated cell and the indirect effect via stimulation of Na^+ reabsorption by the principal cell. With regard to aldosterone's indirect effect (see Chapters 4 and 6), Na^+ reabsorption by the principal cells of the collecting duct is electrogenic and results in the generation of a lumen-negative transepithelial

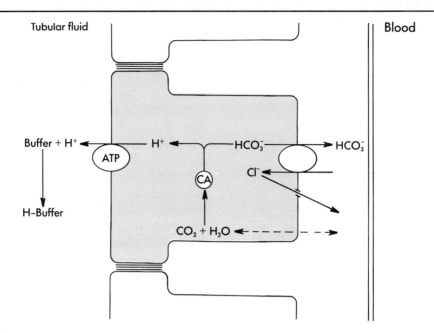

Figure 8-4 ■ General scheme for the excretion of H$^+$ with non-HCO$_3^-$ urinary buffers. The primary urinary buffers are NH$_3$ and HPO$_4^=$ (titratable acid). *CA,* carbonic anhydrase.

voltage. When Na$^+$ reabsorption is stimulated by aldosterone, the magnitude of the lumen-negative voltage is increased. This in turn favors intercalated cell H$^+$ secretion by reducing the electrochemical gradient against which the apical membrane H$^+$-ATPase must pump (the H$^+$-ATPase is electrogenic and thus affected by a voltage gradient). The cell mechanism by which aldosterone directly stimulates intercalated cell H$^+$ secretion is not yet clear. As would be expected, collecting duct H$^+$ secretion is decreased when aldosterone levels are reduced.

■ **FORMATION OF NEW HCO$_3^-$: THE ROLE OF AMMONIA**

As discussed previously, the reabsorption of HCO$_3^-$ is important for the maintenance of acid-base balance. HCO$_3^-$ loss in the urine would decrease the plasma [HCO$_3^-$], and would be equivalent to the addition of H$^+$ to the body. However, HCO$_3^-$ reabsorption alone does not

replenish the HCO$_3^-$ lost during titration of the nonvolatile acids produced by metabolism. To maintain acid-base balance, the kidneys must replace this lost HCO$_3^-$ with *new HCO$_3^-$*. The production of new HCO$_3^-$ is critically dependent upon the availability of urinary buffers. Figure 8-4 illustrates how the titration of these buffers results in the formation of new HCO$_3^-$. Secretion of H$^+$, by combining with a non-HCO$_3^-$ buffer in the tubular fluid, results in the excretion of the H$^+$. HCO$_3^-$ is produced in the cell from the hydration of CO$_2$ and is added to the blood.

As previously noted, the two major urinary buffers are ammonia (NH$_3$/NH$_4^+$) and phosphate (HPO$_4^=$/H$_2$PO$_4^-$). Phosphate is derived solely from the diet. Therefore, the amount excreted in the urine as titratable acid depends on the filtered load minus the amount reabsorbed by the nephron. Ammonia is produced by the kidneys, and its synthesis and subsequent excretion can be regulated in response to the acid-base requirements of the body. Consequently, ammonia is the most important urinary buffer.

The production of new HCO_3^- and the importance of the NH_3/NH_4^+ buffer pair can be summarized for the kidneys as a whole by the following general scheme:

$$\text{Glutamine} \rightarrow NH_4^+ + HCO_3^- \qquad (8\text{-}10)$$

Glutamine is metabolized by the kidneys, and NH_4^+ is excreted into the urine, while HCO_3^- is returned to the systemic circulation to replenish the HCO_3^- lost in the titration of nonvolatile acids. It is important to recognize that the formation of new HCO_3^- by this reaction depends upon the kidney's ability to excrete the NH_4^+ in the urine. If NH_4^+ is not excreted in the urine, but instead enters the systemic circulation, it will titrate plasma HCO_3^-, thus negating the process of new HCO_3^- generation.* The process by which the kidneys excrete NH_4^+ is complex. Figure 8-5 illustrates the essential feature of this process.

NH_4^+ is produced in proximal tubule cells from glutamine. Each glutamine molecule produces two molecules of NH_4^+ and a divalent anion. Metabolism of this anion ultimately provides two molecules of HCO_3^-.

$$\text{Glutamine} \leftrightarrow 2NH_4^+ + \text{anion}^{-2} \leftrightarrow 2HCO_3^- + 2NH_4^+ \quad (8\text{-}11)$$

The HCO_3^- exits the cell across the basolateral membrane and enters the peritubular blood as new HCO_3^-. NH_4^+ exits the cell across the apical membrane and enters the tubular fluid. A major mechanism for the secretion of NH_4^+ into the tubular fluid involves the Na^+-H^+ antiporter, with NH_4^+ substituting for H^+. A large portion of the NH_4^+ secreted by the proximal tubule is reabsorbed by the thick ascending limb of Henle's loop and accumulates in the medullary interstitium. It is then secreted into the tubular fluid by the cells of the collecting duct. The mechanism by which collecting duct NH_4^+ secretion occurs involves the processes of *nonionic diffusion* and *diffusion trapping.*

Ammonia, reabsorbed by the thick ascending limb, accumulates in the medullary interstitial fluid, where it exists as both NH_4^+ and NH_3.* The collecting duct does not have a specific transport mechanism for the secretion of NH_4^+, nor do the cells have a signficant passive permeability to it. However, the cells of the collecting duct are permeable to NH_3, which diffuses from the medullary interstitium into the lumen of the collecting duct. As described previously, H^+ secretion by the collecting duct intercalated cells results in acidification of the luminal fluid (luminal fluid pH as low as 4.0 to 4.5 can be achieved). Consequently, NH_3 diffusing from the medullary interstitium into the collecting duct lumen *(nonionic diffusion)* is protonated to NH_4^+ by the acidic tubular fluid. Because the collecting duct is less permeable to NH_4^+ than to NH_3, NH_4^+ is trapped in the tubule lumen *(diffusion trapping)* and eliminated from the body in the urine.

It is important to note that H^+ secretion by the collecting duct is critical for the excretion of NH_4^+. If collecting duct H^+ secretion is inhibited, the NH_4^+ reabsorbed by the thick ascending limb will not be excreted in the urine; instead, it will be returned to systemic circulation, where it will titrate HCO_3^-. If this occurs, net acid excretion by the kidneys is reduced, and insufficient quantities of new HCO_3^- are added to systemic circulation to replenish what was titrated by the buffering of nonvolatile acids.

---

*The mechanism by which NH_4^+ titrates HCO_3^- is indirect and occurs by the following mechanism:

$$2NH_4^+ \rightarrow \text{urea} + 2H^+ \text{ and}$$
$$2H^+ + 2HCO_3^- \rightarrow 2H_2O + 2CO_2$$

The metabolism of NH_4^+ to urea occurs in the liver.

---

*Ammonia is a weak base that is present as both NH_4^+ and NH_3, with the relative amounts of each species determined by the pKa (pKa = 9).

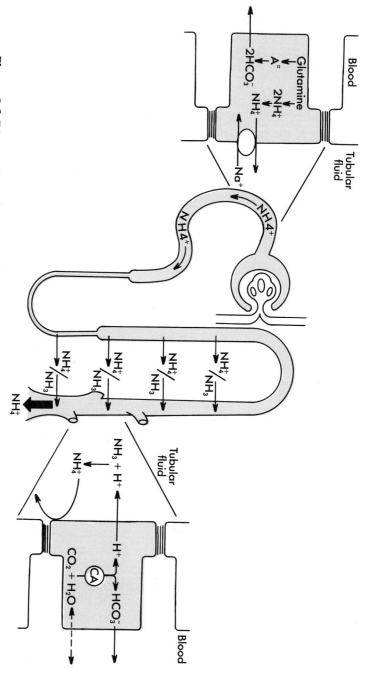

Figure 8-5 ■ Ammonia production and handling by the nephron. Glutamine is metabolized in the proximal tubule to NH_4^+ and HCO_3^-. The NH_4^+ is secreted into the lumen, where it is reabsorbed in the Henle's loop. The NH_4^+ reabsorbed primarily by the thick ascending limb of Henle's loop accumulates in the medullary interstitium where it exists as both NH_4^+ and NH_3. NH_3 diffuses into the tubular fluid of the collecting duct, and H^+ secretion by the collecting duct leads to accumulation of NH_4^+ in the lumen by the processes of nonionic diffusion and diffusion trapping.

An important feature of the NH_4^+ system is that it can be regulated. Alterations in extracellular fluid pH, presumably by affecting intracellular pH, cause changes in NH_4^+ production. During systemic acidosis, the enzymes in the proximal tubule cell, which are responsible for the metabolism of glutamine, are stimulated. This involves the synthesis of new enzyme and requires several days for complete adaptation. With increased levels of this enzyme, NH_4^+ production is increased, thus allowing more H^+ excretion and enhanced production of new HCO_3^-. Conversely, NH_4^+ production is reduced with alkalosis.

Plasma $[K^+]$ also alters NH_4^+ production. With hyperkalemia, NH_4^+ production is inhibited, whereas hypokalemia stimulates production. The mechanism by which plasma K^+ alters NH_4^+ production is not fully understood. It is believed that alterations in plasma $[K^+]$ result in changes in intracellular $[H^+]$ by exchanging H^+ for K^+ (see Chapter 7), and that the change in intracellular pH then controls NH_4^+ production. By this mechanism, exchange of extracellular K^+ for intracellular H^+ during hyperkalemia would raise intracellular pH, thereby inhibiting NH_4^+ production. The opposite would occur during hypokalemia.

■ RESPONSE TO ACID-BASE DISORDERS

The pH of the body fluids is maintained within a very narrow range (pH = 7.40 ± 0.02). *Acidosis* exists when plasma pH falls below 7.40, whereas *alkalosis* exists when the pH is greater than 7.40.* When the acid-base disorder is characterized by a primary change in $[HCO_3^-]$, it is

*In clinical practice, plasma pH values in the range of 7.35 to 7.45 are considered normal. For simplicity, we will consider the single value of 7.40 to represent normal plasma pH, and deviations from this value are deemed abnormal. Similarly, the normal range for Pco_2 is 35 to 45 mm Hg. However, a Pco_2 of 40 mm Hg is used as the normal reference value. Finally, we use a value of 24 mEq/L for normal $[HCO_3^-]$, even though the normal range is from 23 to 25 mEq/L.

termed a *metabolic* disorder. When the disorder is characterized by a primary change in Pco_2, it is termed a *respiratory* disorder.

The body's three general mechanisms to defend against changes in body fluid pH with acid-base disturbances are:
1. Extracellular and intracellular buffering.
2. Adjustments in blood Pco_2 by alterations in the ventilatory rate of the lungs.
3. Adjustments in renal acid excretion.

These mechanisms work in concert to minimize the change in blood pH. However, they do not return blood pH to its normal value by themselves. Restoration of blood pH to its normal value requires correction of the underlying process or processes that produced the acid-base disorder. For example, metabolism of fats in the absence of insulin leads to the accumulation of keto-acids (a nonvolatile acid) in the blood and the development of metabolic acidosis. The acid-base defense mechanisms minimize the fall in pH that occurs with this condition, but normal acid-base balance is not restored until insulin is administered and keto-acid production ceases.

Extracellular and Intracellular Buffering

The first line of defense against acid-base disorders is extracellular and intracellular buffering. The response of the extracellular buffers is virtually instantaneous, whereas cellular buffering is somewhat slower and can take several minutes to complete.

Metabolic disorders resulting from the addition of nonvolatile acids or alkali to the body fluids are buffered primarily in the extracellular fluid and, to a lesser degree, intracellularly. The CO_2/HCO_3^- buffer system is the most important extracellular buffer. Buffering of acid and alkali by this system involves the following reaction:

$$H^+ + HCO_3^- \leftrightarrow H_2CO_3 \leftrightarrow H_2O + CO_2 \quad (8\text{-}12)$$

When nonvolatile acid is added to the body fluids or alkali is lost from the body, the above reaction is driven to the right, HCO_3^- is consumed during the process of buffering the acid load, and plasma $[HCO_3^-]$ is reduced. Thus, metabolic acidosis is characterized by a low pH and $[HCO_3^-]$. Conversely, when nonvolatile alkali is added to the body fluids or acid is lost from the body, the reaction is driven to the left. As a consequence, $[HCO_3^-]$ increases. Thus, metabolic alkalosis is characterized by an increased pH and $[HCO_3^-]$.

Although the CO_2/HCO_3^- buffer system is the primary extracellular buffer, additional extracellular buffering occurs with phosphate and plasma protein.

$$H^+ + HPO_4^- \leftrightarrow H_2PO_4^- \qquad \text{(8-13)}$$
$$H^+ + \text{protein}^- \leftrightarrow \text{H-protein}$$

The combined action of $CO_2/HCO_3^-, HPO_4^-$ and the plasma protein buffering processes accounts for 50% of the buffering of a nonvolatile acid load and 60% to 70% of a nonvolatile alkali load. The remainder of the buffering under these conditions occurs intracellularly.

Intracellular buffering involves the movement of H^+ into cells (during buffering of nonvolatile acid) or the movement of H^+ out of cells (during buffering of nonvolatile alkali).* H^+ is titrated inside the cell by both $HPO_4^-/H_2PO_4^-$ and protein.

With respiratory acid-base disorders, body fluid pH changes as a result of alterations in $[H_2CO_3]$, which is determined directly by the Pco_2 (see Equation 8-1). Virtually all buffering in respiratory acid-base disorders occurs intracellularly. When Pco_2 rises (respiratory acidosis), CO_2 moves into the cell, where it combines

with H_2O to form H_2CO_3. This dissociates to H^+ and HCO_3^-. H^+ is buffered by cellular proteins, and HCO_3^- exits the cell and raises the plasma $[HCO_3^-]$. This process is reversed when Pco_2 is reduced (respiratory alkalosis). Under this condition, the hydration reaction ($H_2O + CO_2 \leftrightarrow H_2CO_3$) is shifted to the left by the decrease in Pco_2. This in turn shifts the dissociation reaction ($H_2CO_3 \leftrightarrow H^+ + HCO_3^-$) to the left, thereby reducing plasma $[HCO_3^-]$.

Respiratory Defense

The lungs are the second line of defense against acid-base disorders. As indicated by the Henderson-Hasselbalch equation, changes in Pco_2 alter the blood pH; an increase in Pco_2 decreases pH, and a decrease in Pco_2 increases pH.

The ventilatory rate is the main determinant of Pco_2. Increased ventilation decreases Pco_2, which normally is 40 mm Hg. With maximal hyperventilation, Pco_2 can be reduced to approximately 10 mm Hg. Conversely, Pco_2 increases with decreased ventilation. Because hypoxia, which is a potent stimulator of ventilation, also develops with hypoventilation, the degree to which Pco_2 can be increased is limited. In a normal individual, Pco_2 generally does not exceed 60 mm Hg. The blood Pco_2 and pH are important regulators of the ventilatory rate. *Chemoreceptors* located in the brain (ventral surface of medulla) and the periphery (carotid and aortic bodies) sense changes in Pco_2 and $[H^+]$, and alter the ventilatory rate. With metabolic acidosis, an increase in $[H^+]$ (decrease in pH) increases the ventilatory rate. Conversely, during metabolic alkalosis, a decrease in $[H^+]$ (increase in pH) leads to a decrease in the ventilatory rate. The respiratory response to metabolic acid-base disturbances may require several hours to complete.

Renal Defense

The third and final line of defense is the kidneys. In response to an alteration in plasma pH

---

*The movement of H^+ into cells is sometimes associated with the release of cellular K^+. Thus hyperkalemia may result with acidosis, while hypokalemia may occur with alkalosis (see Chapter 7). However, the degree of cellular H^+-K^+ exchange depends on the nature of the acid and/or alkali. In general, metabolic acid-base disorders are associated with alterations in K^+, and respiratory disorders are not. Also, metabolic disorders involving organic anions (e.g., lactic acid) have less of an effect on plasma K^+ than mineral acids (e.g., HCl).

and Pco$_2$, the kidneys make appropriate adjustments in the excretion of HCO$_3^-$ and net acid (see Table 8-3). The renal response requires several days to complete.

In the case of acidosis (increase in [H$^+$] or Pco$_2$), secretion of H$^+$ by the nephron is stimulated, and the entire filtered load of HCO$_3^-$ is reabsorbed. The production and excretion of NH$_4^+$ are also stimulated, thus increasing net acid excretion by the kidneys (see Equation 8-9). The new HCO$_3^-$ generated during the process of net acid excretion is returned to the body, and plasma [HCO$_3^-$] increases.

With alkalosis (decrease in [H$^+$] or Pco$_2$), secretion of H$^+$ by the nephron is inhibited and, as a result, net acid excretion and HCO$_3^-$ reabsorption are reduced. HCO$_3^-$ will appear in the urine, thereby reducing plasma [HCO$_3^-$].

■ SIMPLE ACID-BASE DISORDERS

Table 8-4 summarizes the primary alterations and the subsequent defense mechanisms for the various simple acid-base disorders. When considering these disorders, the respiratory and renal defense mechanisms are commonly referred to as compensatory responses. Accordingly, the lungs compensate for metabolic disorders and the kidneys compensate for respiratory disorders.

Metabolic Acidosis

Metabolic acidosis is characterized by low plasma [HCO$_3^-$] and low pH. This condition can develop by the addition of nonvolatile acid to the body (e.g., diabetic ketoacidosis), the loss of nonvolatile alkali (e.g., with diarrhea), or the failure of the kidneys to excrete sufficient net acid to replenish the HCO$_3^-$ used to titrate nonvolatile acids (e.g., renal failure). As described above, buffering of H$^+$ occurs in both the extracellular and intracellular fluid. With a fall in pH, the respiratory centers are stimulted, and the ventilatory rate is increased *(respiratory compensation)*. This reduces Pco$_2$, which further minimizes the fall in plasma pH. In general, there is a 1.2 mm Hg decrease in Pco$_2$ for every 1 mEq/L fall in plasma [HCO$_3^-$]. Thus, if plasma [HCO$_3^-$] were reduced to 14 mEq/L from a normal value of 24 mEq/L, the expected decrease in Pco$_2$ would be 12 mm Hg, and the measured Pco$_2$ would be 28 mm Hg (normal Pco$_2$ = 40 mm Hg).

Finally, renal excretion of net acid is increased. This occurs by eliminating HCO$_3^-$ from the urine (enhanced reabsorption of filtered HCO$_3^-$) and increasing ammonium excretion (enhanced production of new HCO$_3^-$). If the process that initiated the acid-base disturbance is corrected, the enhanced excretion of acid by

Table 8-4 ■ Characteristics of simple acid-base disorders

Disorder	Plasma pH	Primary alteration	Defense mechanism
Metabolic acidosis	↓	↓ Plasma [HCO$_3^-$]	ICF and ECF buffers; Hyperventilation (↓ Pco$_2$)
Metabolic alkalosis	↑	↑ Plasma [HCO$_3^-$]	ICF and ECF buffers; Hypoventilation (↑ Pco$_2$)
Respiratory acidosis	↓	↑ Pco$_2$	ICF buffers; ↑ Renal H$^+$ excretion
Respiratory alkalosis	↑	↓ Pco$_2$	ICF buffers; ↓ Renal H$^+$ excretion

the kidneys will ultimately return the pH and $[HCO_3^-]$ to normal. With correction of the pH, the ventilatory rate will also return to normal.

Metabolic Alkalosis

Metabolic alkalosis is characterized by elevated plasma $[HCO_3^-]$ and pH. This can occur by the addition of nonvolatile alkali to the body (e.g., ingestion of antacids) or, more commonly, from loss of nonvolatile acid (e.g., loss of gastric HCl with vomiting). Buffering occurs in the extracellular and intracellular fluid compartments. The increase in pH inhibits the respiratory centers, and the ventilatory rate is reduced, thus elevating Pco_2 *(respiratory compensation)*. With appropriate respiratory compensation, there is a 0.7 mm Hg increase in Pco_2 for every 1 mEq/L rise in plasma $[HCO_3^-]$.

The renal compensatory response to metabolic alkalosis is an increase in the excretion of HCO_3^- by reducing its reabsorption along the nephron. Normally, this occurs rapidly and effectively. However, when alkalosis occurs in the setting of reduced effective circulating volume (e.g., vomiting), proximal tubule Na^+ reabsorption (and therefore HCO_3^- reabsorption) is enhanced (see Chapter 6). Renal excretion of HCO_3^- and correction of the alkalosis will occur with restoration of a normal effective circulating volume. As occurs with metabolic acidosis, renal excretion of HCO_3^- will eventually return the pH and $[HCO_3^-]$ to normal, provided the underlying cause of the initial disturbance is corrected. With correction of the pH, the ventilatory rate is also returned to normal.

Respiratory Acidosis

Respiratory acidosis is characterized by elevated Pco_2 and reduced plasma pH. It results from decreased gas exchange across the alveoli, either as a result of inadequate ventilation (e.g., drug-induced depression of the respiratory centers) or impaired gas diffusion (e.g., pulmonary edema). In contrast to the metabolic disorders, buffering during respiratory acidosis occurs almost entirely in the intracellular compartment. The increase in Pco_2 and the decrease in pH stimulate both HCO_3^- reabsorption by the kidneys and ammonium excretion *(renal compensation)*. Together, these responses increase net acid excretion and generate new HCO_3^-.

The renal compensatory response takes several days to occur. Consequently, respiratory acid-base disorders are commonly divided into acute and chronic phases. In the acute phase, there has not been sufficient time for the renal compensatory response to occur, and the body relies on intracellular buffering to minimize the change in pH. During this phase, and because of the buffering, there is a 1 mEq/L increase in plasma $[HCO_3^-]$ for every 10 mm Hg rise in Pco_2. In the chronic phase, renal compensation occurs, and there is a 3.5 mEq/L increase in plasma $[HCO_3^-]$ for each 10 mm Hg rise in Pco_2. Correction of the underlying disorder will return Pco_2 to normal, and the renal excretion of acid will decrease to its initial level.

Respiratory Alkalosis

Respiratory alkalosis is characterized by reduced Pco_2 and elevated plasma pH. It results from increased gas exchange in the lungs, usually due to increased ventilation from stimulation of the respiratory centers (e.g., by drugs or CNS disorders). Hyperventilation can also occur as a response to anxiety or fear. As noted, buffering is primarily intracellular. In the acute phase of respiratory alkalosis, it accounts for a 2 mEq/L decrease in plasma $[HCO_3^-]$ for every 10 mm Hg fall in Pco_2. The elevated pH and reduced Pco_2 inhibit HCO_3^- reabsorption by the nephron and reduce ammonium excretion *(renal compensation)*. As a result of these two effects, net acid excretion is reduced. The response takes several days and results in a 5 mEq/ L decrease in plasma $[HCO_3^-]$ for every 10 mm Hg reduction in Pco_2. Correction of the underlying disorder will return Pco_2 to normal, and the renal excretion of acid will increase to its initial level.

■ ANALYSIS OF ACID-BASE DISORDERS

In the clinical setting, analysis of an acid-base disorder is directed at identification of the underlying cause so appropriate therapy can be initiated. The patient's medical history and associated physical findings often provide valuable clues as to the nature and origin of an acid-base disorder. Additionally, analysis of an arterial blood sample is frequently required. Such an analysis is straightforward if approached in a systematic fashion. For example, consider the following data:

$$pH = 7.35 \quad [HCO_3^-] = 16 \text{ mEq/L} \quad P_{CO_2} = 30 \text{ mm Hg}$$

The acid-base disorder represented by these values or any other set of values can be determined by the following three-step approach (see the box below):

1. *Examination of the pH*—By first examining pH, the underlying disorder can be classified as either an acidosis (pH < 7.40) or an alkalosis (pH > 7.40). It should be emphasized that the defense mechanisms of the body cannot correct an acid-base disorder by themselves. Thus, even if the defense mechanisms are completely operative, pH will still indicate the origin of the initial disorder. In the example shown above, the pH of 7.35 indicates an acidosis.

2. *Determination of metabolic vs. respiratory disorder*—Simple acid-base disorders are either metabolic or respiratory. To determine

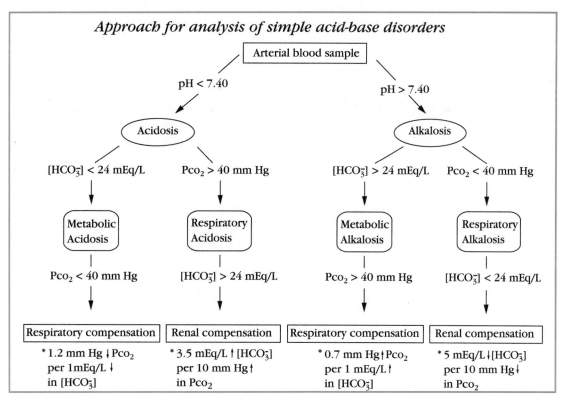

Approach for analysis of simple acid-base disorders

* If the compensatory response is not appropriate, a mixed acid-base disorder should be suspected.

which disorder is present, $[HCO_3^-]$ and Pco_2 must next be examined. As indicated by the Henderson-Hasselbalch equation, a pH value below 7.40 (i.e., acidosis) could be the result of a decrease in $[HCO_3^-]$ (metabolic) or an increase in Pco_2 (respiratory). Alternatively, a pH value above 7.40 (alkalosis) could be the result of an increase in $[HCO_3^-]$ (metabolic) or a decrease in Pco_2 (respiratory). In the above example, $[HCO_3^-]$ is reduced from normal (normal = 23 to 25 mEq/L), as is the Pco_2 (normal = 40 mm Hg). The disorder must therefore be a metabolic acidosis (it cannot be a respiratory acidosis, because Pco_2 is reduced, not increased from normal).

3. *Analysis of compensatory response*—Metabolic disorders result in compensatory changes in ventilation and thus in Pco_2, whereas respiratory disorders result in compensatory changes in renal acid excretion and thus in plasma $[HCO_3^-]$. In an appropriately compensated metabolic acidosis, Pco_2 is decreased, whereas it is elevated with a compensated metabolic alkalosis. With respiratory acidosis, complete compensation results in elevation of $[HCO_3^-]$. Conversely, $[HCO_3^-]$ is reduced in response to a respiratory alkalosis. In the above example, Pco_2 is reduced from normal, and the magnitude of this reduction (10 mm Hg decrease for an 8 mEq/L increase in $[HCO_3^-]$) is as expected. Therefore, the acid-base disorder is a simple metabolic acidosis with appropriate respiratory compensation. If the appropriate compensatory response is not present, a *mixed disorder* should be suspected. A mixed acid-base disorder is simply the presence of two or more underlying causes for the acid-base disturbance. This disorder should be suspected when analysis of the arterial blood gas indicates that appropriate compensation has not occurred. For example, consider the following data:

$$pH = 6.96 \quad [HCO_3^-] = 12 \text{ mEq/L} \quad Pco_2 = 55 \text{ mm Hg}$$

Following the three-step approach outlined above, it is evident that this disturbance is an acidosis that has both a metabolic component ($[HCO_3^-] < 24$ mEq/L) and a respiratory component ($Pco_2 > 40$ mm Hg). Thus, a mixed disorder exists. An example of such a disorder is an individual with a history of chronic pulmonary disease, such as emphysema (chronic respiratory acidosis), who develops an acute gastrointestinal illness with diarrhea. Because diarrhea fluid contains large quantities of HCO_3^-, its loss from the body results in the development of a metabolic acidosis. Note that the finding of a normal pH value with abnormal Pco_2 and $[HCO_3^-]$ values also indicates the presence of a mixed disorder.

■ KEY WORDS AND CONCEPTS

- CO_2/HCO_3^- buffer system
- Carbonic anhydrase
- Henderson-Hasselbalch equation
- Volatile and nonvolatile acid
- Net acid excretion (NAE)
- Titratable acid
- Ammonia/ammonium
- Reabsorption of filtered HCO_3^-
- Formation of new HCO_3^-
- Nonionic diffusion and diffusion trapping of ammonia
- Acidosis (metabolic and respiratory)
- Alkalosis (metabolic and respiratory)
- Chemoreceptors and control of respiration
- Acid-base defense mechanisms
- Respiratory compensation
- Renal compensation
- Simple acid-base disorders
- Mixed acid-base disorders
- Extracellular and intracellular chemical buffers

■ SELF-STUDY PROBLEMS

1. If there were no urinary buffers (e.g., NH_3/NH_4^+ and T.A.), how much urine (L/day)

would the kidneys have to produce in order to excrete net acid equal to the amount of nonvolatile acid produced from metabolism? Assume that nonvolatile acid production is 70 mEq/day, and the minimum urine pH is 4.

2. In the following table, indicate the simple acid-base disorder that exists for the laboratory data given. Use as normal values: pH = 7.40; $[HCO_3^-] = 24$ mEq/L; and $Pco_2 = 40$ mm Hg.

pH	[HCO₃⁻] mEq/L	Pco₂ mm Hg	Disorder
7.34	15	29	_____
7.49	35	48	_____
7.47	14	20	_____
7.34	31	60	_____
7.26	26	60	_____
7.62	20	20	_____
7.09	15	50	_____
7.40	15	25	_____

3. A previously healthy individual develops a gastrointestinal illness with nausea and vomiting. After 12 hours of this illness, the following laboratory data are obtained:

Body weight: 70 kg
Blood pressure: 120/80 mm Hg
Plasma pH: 7.48
Pco₂: 44 mm Hg
Plasma [HCO₃⁻]: 32 mEq/L
Urine pH: 7.5

a. What is the acid-base disorder of this individual? What was its origin?

The illness continues, and 48 hours later the following laboratory data are obtained:

Body weight: 68 kg
Blood pressure: 80/40 mm Hg
Plasma pH: 7.50
Pco₂: 48 mm Hg
Plasma [HCO₃⁻]: 36 mEq/L
Urine pH: 6

b. Has the acid-base disturbance changed? How do you explain the paradoxical decrease in urine pH?

4. What effect would administration of a drug that inhibits carbonic anhydrase be expected to have on urine HCO₃⁻ excretion, and by what mechanism? What type of acid-base disorder could result from the use of this drug?

9 Regulation of Calcium, Magnesium, and Phosphate Balance

■ OBJECTIVES

1. Describe the distribution of Ca^{++}, Mg^{++}, and PO_4^{3-} in the body and their physiological significance.
2. Identify the forms of Ca^{++}, Mg^{++}, and PO_4^{3-} in plasma, and explain the relationship to the amount of Ca^{++}, Mg^{++}, and PO_4^{3-} that is filtered.
3. Explain how the body maintains Ca^{++}, Mg^{++}, and PO_4^{3-} homeostasis and the relative importance of the kidneys vs. the gastrointestinal tract and bone.
4. Describe the hormones and factors that regulate plasma Ca^{++}, Mg^{++}, and PO_4^{3-} levels.
5. Explain the cellular mechanisms of Ca^{++}, Mg^{++}, and PO_4^{3-} reabsorption, and identify the nephron sites at which their excretion is regulated.
6. Describe the hormones that regulate Ca^{++}, Mg^{++}, and PO_4^{3-} excretion.

Ca^{++}, Mg^{++}, and inorganic phosphate (PO_4^{3-})*, are multivalent ions that serve many complex and vital functions. In a normal adult, the renal excretion of these ions is balanced by gastrointestinal absorption. If body stores decline substantially, gastrointestinal absorption, bone resorption, and renal tubular reabsorption increase to return body stores to normal levels. During growth and pregnancy, intestinal absorption exceeds urinary excretion, and these ions accumulate in newly formed fetal tissue and bone. In contrast, bone disease (e.g., osteoporosis) or a decrease in lean body mass increases urinary mineral loss without changing intestinal absorption. Under these conditions, there is a net loss of Ca^{++}, Mg^{++}, and PO_4^{3-} from the body.

From this brief introduction, it is evident that *the kidneys, in conjunction with the gastrointestinal tract and bone, play a major role in maintaining Ca^{++}, Mg^{++}, and PO_4^{3-} homeostasis.* Accordingly, this chapter discusses how Ca^{++}, Mg^{++}, and PO_4^{3-} are handled by the kidneys, with an emphasis on the hormones and factors that regulate urinary excretion.

■ Ca^{++}

Ca^{++} ions play a major role in many processes, including bone formation, cell division

---

*At physiological pH phosphate exists as $HPO_4^{=}$ and $H_2PO_4^{-}$ (pK = 6.8). For simplicity, we collectively refer to these ion species as PO_4^{3-}.

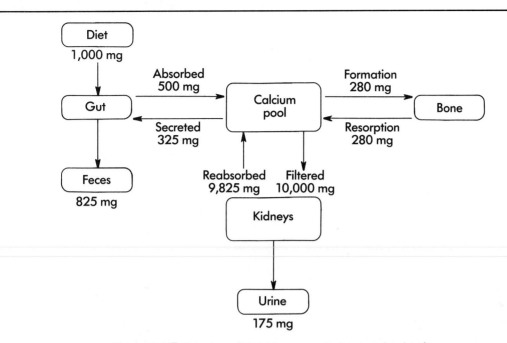

Figure 9-1 ▪ Overview of Ca^{++} homeostasis. See text for details.

Table 9-1 ▪ Body content and distribution of Ca^{++}, Mg^{++}, and PO_4^{3-}

			Compartment	
Ion	Body content	Bone	Intracellular	Extracellular
Ca^{++}	1,300 gm	99%	1%	0.10%
Mg^{++}	26 gm	54%	45%	1.00%
PO_4^{3-}	700 gm	86%	14%	0.03%

and growth, blood coagulation, hormone-response coupling, and electrical stimulus-response coupling (e.g., muscle contraction and neurotransmitter release). Ninety-nine percent of Ca^{++} is stored in bone, 1% is found in the intracellular fluid, and 0.1% is located in the extracellular fluid (Table 9-1). The total $[Ca^{++}]$ in plasma is approximately 5 mEq/L, and its concentration is normally maintained within very narrow limits. A low $[Ca^{++}]$ increases the excitability of nerve and muscle cells. Diseases that lower plasma $[Ca^{++}]$ cause hypocalcemic tetany, which is characterized by skeletal muscle spasms. Hypercalcemia causes cardiac arrhythmias and decreased neuromuscular excitability.

Overview of Ca^{++} Homeostasis

The maintenance of Ca^{++} homeostasis is a function of two variables: the total amount of Ca^{++} in the body and the distribution of Ca^{++} between the intracellular and extracellular fluid compartments. As illustrated in Figure 9-1, total body Ca^{++} is determined by the relative amounts of Ca^{++} absorbed by the gastrointestinal tract and excreted by the kidneys. Ca^{++} absorption by the gastrointestinal tract occurs by an active, carrier-mediated transport mechanism that is stimulated by 1,25-dihydroxyvitamin D_3 (1,25($OH)_2D_3$). Net Ca^{++} absorption is normally 175 mg/day, but it can increase to 600 mg/day when 1,25($OH)_2D_3$ levels rise. Ca^{++} excretion by the kidneys is equal to the amount absorbed by the gastrointestinal tract (175 mg/day) and changes parallel to the absorption of Ca^{++} by the gastrointestinal tract. Thus, Ca^{++} balance is maintained, because the amount of Ca^{++} ingested in an average diet (1,000 mg/day) is equal to the amount lost in the feces (825 mg/day: the fraction that escapes absorption by the gastrointestinal tract) plus the amount excreted in the urine (175 mg/day).

The other variable controlling Ca^{++} homeostasis is its distribution between bone and the extracellular fluid. Parathyroid hormone (PTH) and 1,25($OH)_2D_3$ are the most important hormones controlling this variable and thereby regulate plasma $[Ca^{++}]$. Secretion of PTH by the parathyroid glands is stimulated by a decline in plasma $[Ca^{++}]$ (i.e., hypocalcemia). PTH increases plasma $[Ca^{++}]$ by:

1. Stimulating bone resorption.
2. Increasing Ca^{++} reabsorption by the kidneys.
3. Stimulating the production of 1,25($OH)_2D_3$, which in turn increases Ca^{++} absorption by the gastrointestinal tract and stimulates bone resorption.

Hypercalcemia reduces PTH secretion, which leads to actions opposite those described above.

Ca^{++} Transport Along the Nephron

As shown in Table 9-2, approximately 50% of Ca^{++} in plasma is ionized, 45% is bound to plasma proteins, primarily albumin, and 5% is complexed to several anions, including HCO_3^-, citrate, PO_4^{3-} and $SO_4^=$. The pH of the plasma influences this distribution. Acidosis increases the percentage of ionized Ca^{++}, at the expense of protein-bound Ca^{++}, whereas alkalosis decreases the percentage of ionized Ca^{++}, again by altering protein-bound Ca^{++}. The Ca^{++} available for filtration is the ionized fraction and that complexed with anions. Thus, about 55% of the Ca^{++} in the plasma is available for glomerular filtration.

Normally, 99% of the filtered Ca^{++} is reabsorbed by the nephron, of which 70% is reabsorbed by the proximal tubule (Figure 9-2). Another 20% is reabsorbed in Henle's loop (mainly the thick ascending limb), 5% to 10% is reabsorbed by the distal tubule, and <5% is reabsorbed by the collecting duct. About 1% (8.6 mEq/day or 175 mg/day) is excreted in the urine. This is equal to the net amount absorbed daily by the gastrointestinal tract.

Table 9-2 ■ Forms of Ca^{++}, Mg^{++}, and PO_4^{3-} in plasma

Ion	mEq/L	Percentage of total		
		Ionized	Protein-bound	Complexed
Ca^{++}	5 mEq/L	50%	45%	5%
Mg^{++}	2 mEq/L	55%	30%	15%
PO_4^{3-}	2 mEq/L	84%	10%	6%

Ca^{++} and Mg^{++} are bound (i.e., complexed) to various anions in the plasma, including HCO_3^-, citrate, PO_4^{3-}, and $SO_4^=$. PO_4^{3-} is complexed to various cations, including Na^+ and K^+.

Cellular Mechanisms of Ca^{++} Reabsorption

Ca^{++} reabsorption by the proximal tubule occurs by transcellular and paracellular pathways (Figure 9-3). Ca^{++} reabsorption across the cellular pathway, which accounts for one third of proximal reabsorption, occurs in two steps. Ca^{++} diffuses across the apical membrane into the cell down its electrochemical gradient. This gradient is exceptionally steep, because the cell Ca^{++} concentration is only 0.2 µEq/L, some 10,000 times less than its concentration in the tubular fluid (3 mEq/L). The cell interior is electrically negative with respect to the luminal side of the apical membrane, which also favors Ca^{++} entry into the cell. Ca^{++} is extruded across the basolateral membrane against its electrochem-

ical gradient, making extrusion an active process. The mechanism for the active extrusion of Ca^{++} has not been identified, but could occur by a Ca^{++}-ATPase or $3Na^{+}$-Ca^{++} antiporter. Two thirds of Ca^{++} is reabsorbed across the paracellular pathway by solvent drag along the length of the proximal tubule and, in the second half of the proximal tubule, by passive diffusion, due to the lumen-positive transepithelial voltage.

Ca^{++} reabsorption by Henle's loop is restricted to the thick ascending limb. Ca^{++} is reabsorbed via cellular and paracellular routes by mechanisms similar to those described for the proximal tubule. The difference is that Ca^{++} is not reabsorbed by solvent drag in this segment (recall that the thick ascending limb is impermeable to water). In both the proximal tubule and thick ascending limb, Ca^{++} and Na^{+} reabsorption parallel each other. This is due to the significant component of Ca^{++} reabsorption that occurs by passive paracellular mechanisms secondary to Na^{+} reabsorption and the generation of the lumen-positive transepithelial voltages in these segments. Therefore, *changes in Na^{+} reabsorption will alter Ca^{++} reabsorption in parallel by the proximal tubule and thick ascending limb.*

In the distal tubule and collecting duct, where the voltage in the tubular fluid is electrically negative with respect to the blood, Ca^{++} reabsorption is entirely active because it is reabsorbed against its electrochemical gradient. The mechanisms of Ca^{++} reabsorption by these segments have not been elucidated. *Because the reabsorption of Ca^{++} and Na^{+} by the early distal tubule and collecting duct are independent and differentially regulated, urinary Ca^{++} and Na^{+} excretion do not always change in parallel.*

Regulation of Ca^{++} Excretion

The hormones and factors regulating urinary Ca^{++} excretion are summarized in the box on p. 144. *Parathyroid hormone (PTH) exerts the*

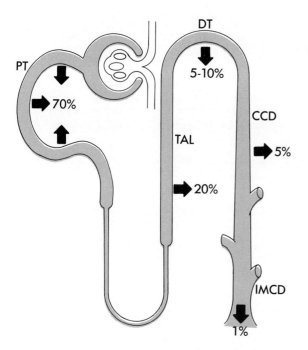

Figure 9-2 ■ Transport pattern of Ca^{++} along the nephron. Percentages refer to the amount of the filtered Ca^{++} reabsorbed by each nephron segment. Approximately 1% of the filtered Ca^{++} is excreted. *PT,* proximal tubule; *TAL,* thick ascending limb; *DT,* distal tubule; *CCD,* cortical collecting duct; *IMCD,* inner medullary collecting duct.

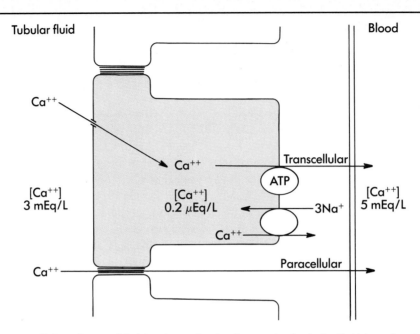

Figure 9-3 ■ Cellular scheme of Ca^{++} reabsorption by the proximal tubule. Ca^{++} is reabsorbed by transcellular and paracellular routes. The mechanism of Ca^{++} diffusion into the cell across the apical membrane has not been characterized, but is likely to occur via Ca^{++} channels.

most powerful control on renal Ca^{++} excretion. This hormone stimulates overall Ca^{++} reabsorption. Although PTH inhibits fluid and therefore Ca^{++} reabsorption by the proximal tubule, it dramatically stimulates Ca^{++} reabsorption by the thick ascending limb of Henle's loop and the distal tubule. As a result, urinary Ca^{++} excretion declines. An increase in plasma [PO$_4^{3-}$] (e.g., increased dietary intake of PO$_4^{3-}$ or ingestion of large amounts of PO$_4^{3-}$-containing antacids) increases PTH levels and thereby decreases Ca^{++} excretion, whereas a decline in plasma [PO$_4^{3-}$] (e.g., dietary PO$_4^{3-}$ depletion) has the opposite effect.

Changes in the extracellular fluid volume alter Ca^{++} excretion mainly by affecting Na$^+$ and fluid reabsorption in the proximal tubule. Contraction of the extracellular fluid volume increases Na$^+$ and water reabsorption by the proximal tubule, thereby enhancing Ca^{++} reabsorption.

Accordingly, urinary Ca^{++} excretion declines. Expansion of the extracellular fluid volume has the opposite effect.

Acidosis increases Ca^{++} excretion, whereas alkalosis decreases it. The regulation of Ca^{++} reabsorption by pH occurs in the distal tubule by an unknown mechanism.

Finally, 1,25(OH)$_2$D$_3$ increases Ca^{++} reabsorption by the distal tubule, thereby decreasing Ca^{++} excretion.

■ Mg^{++}

Mg^{++} is the second most common intracellular electrolyte. It has many biochemical roles, including activation of enzymes and regulation of protein synthesis. It is also important for bone formation. The distribution of Mg^{++} in the body and its forms in plasma are summarized in Tables 9-1 and 9-2. Of Mg^{++} in the body, 54% is located in bone, 45% in the

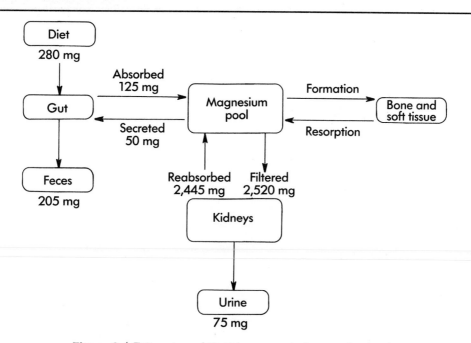

Figure 9-4 ▪ Overview of Mg^{++} homeostasis. See text for details.

<table>
<tr><td colspan="2" align="center">*Hormones and factors influencing urinary Ca^{++} excretion*</td></tr>
<tr><td>**Increase Excretion**</td><td>**Decrease Excretion**</td></tr>
<tr><td>Decrease in [PTH]</td><td>Increase in [PTH]</td></tr>
<tr><td>ECF expansion</td><td>ECF contraction</td></tr>
<tr><td>PO_4^{3-} depletion</td><td>PO_4^{3-} loading</td></tr>
<tr><td>Metabolic acidosis</td><td>Metabolic alkalosis</td></tr>
<tr><td></td><td>$1,25(OH)_2D_3$</td></tr>
</table>

intracellular fluid, and 1% in the extracellular fluid. Plasma $[Mg^{++}]$ is about 2.0 mEq/L. Approximately 30% of Mg^{++} is protein-bound and therefore unavailable for ultrafiltration by the glomerulus. The Mg^{++} that is filtered consists of an ionized fraction (55%) and a nonionized component (15%) that is complexed to HCO_3^-, citrate, PO_4^{3-}, and $SO_4^=$. Accordingly, the Mg^{++} concentration in the glomerular ultrafiltrate is 30% less than the Mg^{++} concentration in plasma.

Overview of Mg^{++} Homeostasis

Figure 9-4 is a general scheme of Mg^{++} homeostasis. As with Ca^{++}, the maintenance of $[Mg^{++}]$ in body fluids is a function of two variables: the total amount of Mg^{++} in the body and the distribution of Mg^{++} between the intracellular and extracellular fluid compartments. Total body Mg^{++} is determined by the relative amount of net Mg^{++} absorption by the gastrointestinal tract and excretion by the kidneys. The kidneys maintain body Mg^{++} balance by their ability to excrete in the urine an amount of Mg^{++} equal to that absorbed by the gastrointestinal tract (i.e., 75 mg/day). Although the gastrointestinal absorption of Mg^{++} is not regulated as closely as that for Ca^{++}, when dietary intake is restricted, intestinal absorption rises. The hormones and factors responsible for the regulation of intestinal Mg^{++} absorption are unknown.

The other variable regulating Mg^{++} homeostasis is the distribution of Mg^{++} between the intracellular and extracellular fluid. The hormones and factors regulating this variable have not been identified.

Mg^{++} Transport Along the Nephron

The kidneys play a vital role in Mg^{++} homeostasis by excreting 3% of the filtered Mg^{++}. Mg^{++} reabsorption by the nephron exhibits a T_m that is increased by PTH. The pattern of Mg^{++} transport along the nephron is shown in Figure 9-5. Approximately 30% of the filtered Mg^{++} is reabsorbed by the proximal tubule. The thick ascending limb of Henle's loop is the major site of Mg^{++} transport, reabsorbing 65% of the filtered Mg^{++}. Reabsorption is passive and driven by the lumen-positive transepithelial voltage across this nephron segment. *Alterations in urinary Mg^{++} excretion usually arise from changes in Mg^{++} reabsorption by the thick ascending limb.* Very little Mg^{++} is reabsorbed by the distal tubule and collecting duct (<2%). The mechanisms of Mg^{++} transport along the nephron are poorly understood; however, reabsorption is thought to be passive and driven by the lumen-positive transepithelial voltage in the late proximal tubule and thick ascending limb.

Regulation of Mg^{++} Excretion

The box on p. 147 summarizes the major hormones and factors that regulate Mg^{++} excretion. Hypercalcemia, hypermagnesemia, extra-

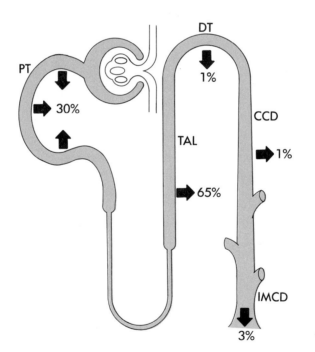

Figure 9-5 ■ Transport pattern of Mg^{++} along the nephron. Mg^{++} is reabsorbed mainly by the proximal tubule and the thick ascending limb of Henle's loop. Percentages refer to the amount of the filtered Mg^{++} reabsorbed by each nephron segment. Approximately 3% of the filtered Mg^{++} is excreted. *PT,* proximal tubule; *TAL,* thick ascending limb; *DT,* distal tubule; *CCD,* cortical collecting duct; *IMCD,* inner medullary collecting duct.

cellular fluid volume expansion, acidosis, and a decrease in PTH levels cause an increase in excretion. Hypocalcemia, hypomagnesemia, extracellular volume contraction, alkalosis, and an increase in PTH levels result in decreased excretion. All of these regulatory influences have a direct effect on Na^+ reabsorption and thus the transepithelial voltage. By changing the transepithelial voltage, these regulatory influences modulate Mg^{++} reabsorption across the paracellular pathway. Also, alterations in extracellular fluid volume regulate Na^+ and water reabsorption, thus influencing Mg^{++} reabsorption by affecting solvent drag and the paracellular diffusion of Mg^{++}.

■ PO_4^{3-}

PO_4^{3-} is an important component of many organic molecules, including DNA, RNA, ATP, and intermediates of metabolic pathways. It is also a major constituent of bone. Its concentration in plasma is an important determinant of bone formation and resorption. In addition, urinary PO_4^{3-} is an important buffer (titratable acid) for the maintenance of acid-base balance. Eighty-six percent of PO_4^{3-} is located in bone, 14% in intracellular fluid and 0.03% in extracellular fluid (Table 9-1). Plasma $[PO_4^{3-}]$ is 2 mEq/L. The forms of PO_4^{3-} in plasma are summarized in Table 9-2. Approximately 10% of the PO_4^{3-} in plasma is protein-bound and therefore unavailable for ultrafiltration by the glomerulus.

Hormones and factors influencing urinary Mg^{++} excretion

Increase Excretion	Decrease Excretion
Hypercalcemia	Hypocalcemia
Hypermagnesemia	Hypomagnesemia
ECF expansion	ECF contraction
Decrease of [PTH]	Increase of [PTH]
Acidosis	Alkalosis

Accordingly, the $[PO_4^{3-}]$ in the ultrafiltrate is 10% less than that in plasma.

Overview of PO_4^{3-} Homeostasis

Figure 9-6 is a general scheme of PO_4^{3-} homeostasis. The maintenance of PO_4^{3-} homeostasis is a function of two variables: the amount of PO_4^{3-} in the body and the distribution of PO_4^{3-} between the intracellular and extracellular fluid compartments. Total body PO_4^{3-} is determined by the relative amount of PO_4^{3-} absorbed by the gastrointestinal tract vs. the amount excreted by the kidneys. PO_4^{3-} absorption by the gastrointestinal tract occurs by active and passive mechanisms. It increases as dietary PO_4^{3-} rises and is stimulated by $1,25(OH)_2D_3$. Despite changes in PO_4^{3-} intake (between 800 and 1,500 mg/day), total body PO_4^{3-} balance is maintained by the kidneys, which excrete in the urine an amount of PO_4^{3-} equal to that absorbed by the gastrointestinal tract. Thus, *the kidneys play a vital role in maintaining PO_4^{3-} homeostasis.*

The second variable maintaining PO_4^{3-} homeostasis is the distribution of PO_4^{3-} between bone and the intracellular and extracellular fluid compartments. The release of PO_4^{3-} from intracellular stores is stimulated by the same hormones that release Ca^{++} from this pool: PTH and $1,25(OH)_2D_3$. Thus, the release of PO_4^{3-} is always accompanied by a release of Ca^{++}. The kidneys also significantly contribute to the regulation of plasma $[PO_4^{3-}]$. Consider the PO_4^{3-} titration curve, illustrated in Figure 9-7. Recalling the glucose titration curve presented in Chapter 3, it should be evident that the tubular mechanisms for PO_4^{3-} reabsorption share many properties with glucose transport. These include a T_m, splay, and a threshold. However, the titration curves for glucose and PO_4^{3-} are significantly different in other respects. First, the T_m for PO_4^{3-} is only slightly above the normal filtered load. Hence, a small increase in plasma $[PO_4^{3-}]$ increases the filtered load, such that the

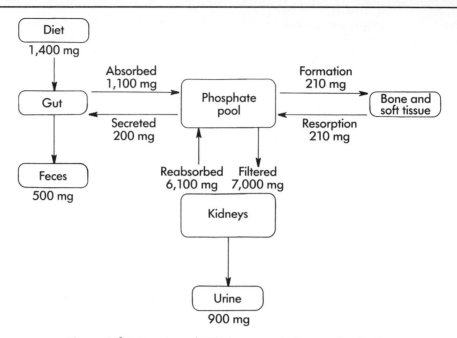

Figure 9-6 ■ Overview of PO$_4^{3-}$ homeostasis. See text for details.

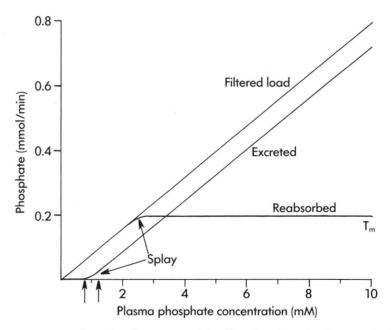

Figure 9-7 ■ Titration curve for PO$_4^{3-}$. The amount of the filtered PO$_4^{3-}$ reabsorbed is calculated as the difference between the amount filtered minus the amount excreted. The arrows on the x-axis indicate the normal range of plasma [PO$_4^{3-}$] (normal plasma [PO$_4^{3-}$] is 0.8 to 1.2 mM or 2.4 to 3.6 mEq/L). T$_m$, transport maximum.

T_m is exceeded and urinary PO_4^{3-} excretion rises (Figure 9-7). This in turn causes plasma $[PO_4^{3-}]$ to fall. Accordingly, *the kidneys regulate plasma $[PO_4^{3-}]$*. In contrast, because the T_m for glucose is considerably above its normal filtered load, small changes in plasma glucose do not change glucose excretion or plasma glucose concentration. Thus, the kidneys do not regulate plasma glucose levels in healthy individuals.

A second unique aspect of the PO_4^{3-} titration curve is that the T_m for PO_4^{3-} is variable and regulated by dietary PO_4^{3-} intake. A high PO_4^{3-} diet decreases the T_m, and a low PO_4^{3-} diet increases it. This effect of dietary PO_4^{3-} intake on the T_m is independent of changes in PTH levels. In contrast, the T_m for glucose is relatively stable.

PO_4^{3-} Transport Along the Nephron

Figure 9-8 illustrates the transport pattern of PO_4^{3-} along the nephron. The proximal tubule reabsorbs 80% of the PO_4^{3-} filtered by the glomerulus, and the distal tubule reabsorbs 10%. In contrast, Henle's loop and the collecting duct reabsorb negligible amounts of PO_4^{3-}. Therefore, 10% of the filtered load of PO_4^{3-} is excreted.

PO_4^{3-} reabsorption by the proximal tubule occurs mainly, if not exclusively, by a transcellular route. As shown in Figure 9-9, PO_4^{3-} uptake across the apical membrane occurs via a $2Na^+$-PO_4^{3-} symport mechanism. PO_4^{3-} exit across the basolateral membrane occurs by a PO_4^{3-}-anion antiporter. The cellular mechanisms of PO_4^{3-} reabsorption by the distal tubule and cortical collecting duct have not been characterized.

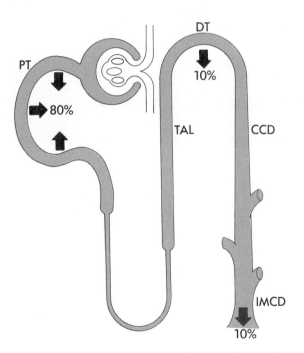

Figure 9-8 ■ Transport pattern of PO_4^{3-} along the nephron. PO_4^{3-} is reabsorbed primarily by the proximal tubule and distal tubule. Percentages refer to the amount of the filtered PO_4^{3-} reabsorbed by each nephron segment. Approximately 10% of the filtered PO_4^{3-} is excreted. *PT,* proximal tubule; *TAL,* thick ascending limb; *DT,* distal tubule; *CCD,* cortical collecting duct; *IMCD,* inner medullary collecting duct.

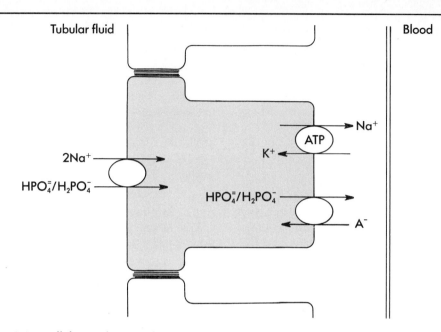

Figure 9-9 ■ Cellular mechanism of PO_4^{3-} reabsorption by the proximal tubule. See the text for details.

Hormones and factors influencing urinary PO_4^{3-} excretion	
Increase Excretion	**Decrease Excretion**
Increase of [PTH]	Decrease of [PTH]
PO_4^{3-} loading	PO_4^{3-} depletion
ECF expansion	ECF contraction
Glucocorticoids	
Acidosis	Alkalosis

Regulation of PO_4^{3-} Excretion

The major hormones and factors that regulate PO_4^{3-} excretion are summarized in the box above. All act on the proximal tubule to either stimulate or inhibit PO_4^{3-} reabsorption. *PTH is the most important hormone controlling PO_4^{3-} excretion.* PTH increases cAMP production and inhibits PO_4^{3-} reabsorption by the proximal tubule. Dietary PO_4^{3-} intake also regulates PO_4^{3-} excretion by mechanisms unrelated to changes in PTH levels. PO_4^{3-} loading increases excretion, whereas PO_4^{3-} depletion decreases excretion. Changes in dietary PO_4^{3-} intake modulate PO_4^{3-} transport by altering the transport rate of each $2Na^+-PO_4^{3-}$ symporter without changing the number of transporters.

Extracellular fluid volume also affects PO_4^{3-} excretion: volume expansion increases excretion, and volume contraction decreases it. Glucocorticoids increase the excretion of PO_4^{3-}. By inhibiting proximal tubular PO_4^{3-} reabsorption, glucocorticoids increase the delivery of PO_4^{3-} to the distal tubule and collecting duct. This enables these segments to secrete more H^+ and thereby generate more HCO_3^- (PO_4^{3-} is an important urinary buffer and is termed a titratable acid). For example, in the absence of glucocorticoids (e.g., Addison's disease), PO_4^{3-} excretion is depressed, as is the kidneys' ability to excrete titratable acid and generate new HCO_3^-. Acid-base balance also influences PO_4^{3-} excretion, with acidosis increasing and alkalosis decreasing excretion.

■ KEY WORDS AND CONCEPTS

- Ca^{++} homeostasis
- PTH
- 1,25-dihydroxyvitamin D_3 ($1,25(OH)_2D_3$)
- Hypocalcemia
- Hypercalcemia
- Regulation of renal Ca^{++} excretion
- Mg^{++} homeostasis
- Regulation of renal Mg^{++} excretion
- PO_4^{3-} homeostasis
- PO_4^{3-} titration curve
- PTH is the most important regulator of PO_4^{3-} excretion.

■ SELF-STUDY PROBLEMS

1. How is Ca^{++} reabsorption in the proximal tubule dependent on Na^+ reabsorption? What would happen to Ca^{++} excretion if a subject was given a diuretic, such as mannitol, that inhibits sodium and water reabsorption by the proximal tubule?

2. What effect would furosemide, an inhibitor of Na^+ reabsorption by the thick ascending limb of Henle's loop, have on urinary Ca^{++} excretion?

3. What would happen to PO_4^{3-} excretion if plasma $[PO_4^{3-}]$ was increased from 2 to 3 mEq/L?

10 Physiology of Diuretic Action

■ OBJECTIVES

1. Explain the effects of diuretic agents on Na^+ handling by the kidneys and on the extracellular fluid volume.
2. Explain the importance of the proximal tubule organic anion and organic cation secretory systems to the delivery of diuretics into the lumen of the nephron.

3. Define the nephron sites at which the various classes of diuretics act and the specific transport mechanisms inhibited.
4. Describe the effects of diuretics on the renal handling of K^+, Ca^{++}, HCO_3^-, Mg^{++}, PO_4^{3-}, and solute-free water.

Diuretics, as the name implies, cause an increase in urine output. It is important, however, to distinguish this diuresis from that which occurs following the ingestion of large volumes of water. In the latter case, the urine is comprised largely of water, and solute excretion is not increased. In contrast, diuretics result in increased excretion of both solute and water.

All diuretics have as their common mode of action the inhibition of Na^+ reabsorption by the nephron. Consequently, they cause an increase in Na^+ excretion, termed *natriuresis*. The effects of diuretics, however, are not limited to Na^+ handling. The renal handling of many other solutes is also influenced, usually as a consequence of alterations in Na^+ transport.

This chapter reviews the cellular mechanisms of action of the various diuretics and the nephron sites at which they act. In addition to examining their effects on Na^+ handling by the nephron, their effects on the renal handling of

other solutes (K^+, Ca^{++}, Mg^{++}, PO_4^{3-}, and HCO_3^-) and water are also explained.

■ GENERAL PRINCIPLES OF DIURETIC ACTION

The primary action of diuretics is to increase the excretion of Na^+. As described in Chapter 6, alterations in Na^+ excretion by the kidneys result in alterations in the volume of the extracellular fluid (ECF) compartment. Consequently, diuretics decrease the volume of the ECF. Indeed, diuretics are commonly given in clinical situations in which the ECF compartment is expanded, with the intent of reducing its volume.

The effects of diuretic administration, although generally predictable for a particular class of diuretics, can be quite variable. Several factors are important in determining the overall effect of a particular diuretic:

1. The nephron segment where the diuretic acts

2. The response of nephron segments distal to the site of action of the diuretic
3. The delivery of sufficient quantities of the diuretic to its site of action
4. The volume of the ECF

Sites of Action of Diuretics

Diuretics act on specific renal tubule transporters. Consequently, a diuretic's site of action is determined by the localization of these transporters along the nephron. Figure 10-1 depicts the nephron sites at which the different classes of diuretics act. The osmotic diuretics act along the proximal tubule and thin descending limb of Henle's loop. The carbonic anhydrase inhibitors act primarily in the proximal tubule. The thick ascending limb of Henle's loop is the site of action of the loop diuretics. The early portion of the distal tubule is the site of action of the

thiazide diuretics, and the K+-sparing diuretics act on the late portion of the distal tubule and the cortical collecting duct.

The site of action of a diuretic in turn determines the magnitude of the associated natriuresis. The effect diuretics have on the handling of solutes other than Na+ is also dependent upon the site of action. Examples illustrating this point are given in subsequent sections.

Response of More Distal Nephron Segments

When a diuretic inhibits Na+ reabsorption at one nephron site, it causes the increased delivery of Na+ and water to more distal segments. The function of these segments and their ability or inability to handle this increased load ultimately determines the overall effect of the diuretic on urinary excretion. Examples of this

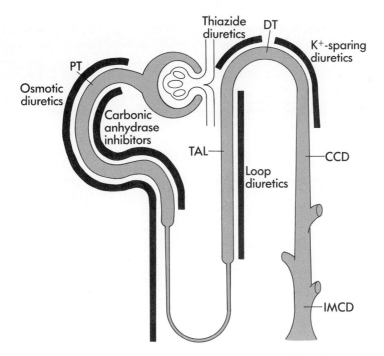

Figure 10-1 ■ Sites of action of diuretics along the nephron. *PT*, proximal tubule; *TAL*, thick ascending limb; *DT*, distal tubule; *CCD*, cortical collecting duct; *IMCD*, inner medullary collecting duct.

are considered in detail below with each of the various diuretics.

Adequate Delivery of Diuretics to Their Site of Action

The effect of a diuretic on Na^+ excretion is also dependent upon the delivery of adequate quantities of the drug to its site of action. With the exception of the aldosterone antagonists, which act intracellulary, diuretic agents act from the lumen of the nephron (carbonic anhydrase inhibitors have both a luminal and intracellular site of action). Diuretics gain access to the lumen by glomerular filtration and through secretion by the *organic anion* and *organic cation secretory systems* located in the proximal tubule (see Chapter 4). Thus, the effect of a diuretic can be blunted if, for example, it is administered with another drug that competes for the same secretory mechanism.

Volume of the ECF

Finally, the effect of a diuretic is dependent upon the ECF volume. As described in Chapter 6, when the ECF volume is decreased, GFR is reduced, thereby reducing the filtered load of Na^+. In addition, Na^+ reabsorption by the proximal tubule is enhanced. For example, the effect of a diuretic that acts on the distal tubule would be blunted if administered in the setting of reduced ECF volume. Under this condition, the decreased GFR (i.e., decreased filtered load of Na^+), together with enhanced Na^+ reabsorption by the proximal tubule, would result in the delivery of a smaller quantity of Na^+ to the distal tubule. Thus, even if the diuretic completely inhibited Na^+ reabsorption in the distal tubule, the associated natriuresis would be less than that with a normal ECF volume.

The dependence of diuretic-induced natriuresis on ECF volume also explains why the effect of a diuretic is self-limited. As illustrated in Figure 10-2, administration of a diuretic to an individual with fixed Na^+ intake results in a short-lived natriuresis. This transient response reflects the fact that, by increasing Na^+ excretion, the diuretic reduces the volume of the ECF (detected as a decrease in body weight). Such a fall in ECF volume decreases GFR and increases proximal tubule reabsorption. These ef-

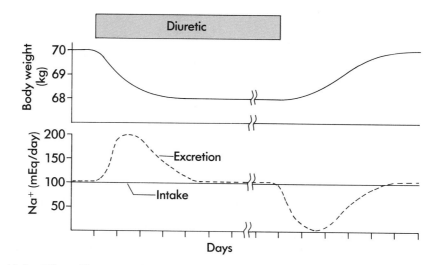

Figure 10-2 ■ Effect of long-term diuretic therapy on renal Na^+ excretion. Because of diuretic-induced natriuresis the extracellular fluid volume is reduced. This is detected as a decrease in body weight.

fects in turn limit the natriuretic response, as described above. After a short period (usually several days), the individual reaches a new steady state, during which Na^+ intake again equals excretion. However, the volume of the ECF is decreased. When diuretic therapy is discontinued, renal Na^+ excretion is reduced. After a period of positive Na^+ balance, during which the volume of the ECF is returned to normal (return of body weight to original value), a new steady state is again achieved.

The concept of *steady state* deserves special emphasis. Normally, individuals are in steady-state balance with regard to solute (e.g., Na^+) and water, with intake equaling excretion. Administration of a diuretic temporarily disrupts this balance by increasing excretion, and a negative balance exists. However, excretion cannot exceed intake indefinitely, and a new steady-state is eventually achieved. In this new steady state, intake and excretion are again balanced, but ECF volume is reduced. When attempting to analyze the effects of diuretic therapy, consideration must be given to whether the individual is in the acute phase (i.e., negative balance) or chronic phase (i.e., steady state). In general, when an individual is continued on a diuretic for several days or longer, a new steady state will have been achieved, and ECF volume will be reduced from what it was prior to diuretic administration.

■ MECHANISMS OF ACTION OF DIURETICS

Osmotic Diuretics

Osmotic diuretics, as the name implies, are agents that inhibit the reabsorption of solute and water by altering osmotic forces along the nephron. The best example of an exogenous osmotic diuretic is the sugar mannitol. When present in abnormally high concentrations, endogenous substances, such as glucose (i.e., in diabetes mellitus) and urea (i.e., in uremia), can also act as osmotic diuretics.

Osmotic diuretics (e.g., mannitol) gain access to the tubular fluid by glomerular filtration. Because they are not reabsorbed or only poorly reabsorbed, they remain within the lumen, where they can exert an osmotic pressure that inhibits tubular fluid reabsorption. Osmotic diuretics affect fluid reabsorption in those segments that are highly permeable to water (i.e., the proximal tubule and thin descending limb of Henle's loop). Because of the large volumes of filtrate reabsorbed in the proximal tubule (60% to 70% of the filtered load), this nephron site is the most important when considering the action of osmotic diuretics.

As described in Chapter 4, reabsorption of tubular fluid by the proximal tubule is essentially an isosmotic process (i.e., the osmolality of the reabsorbed fluid is slightly hyperosmotic to tubular fluid). Solute (primarily NaCl) is actively reabsorbed by the proximal tubule cells. This sets up a small osmotic pressure difference across the tubule, with the lumen being 3 to 5 mOsm/kg H_2O hyposmotic with respect to the interstitial fluid. Given the high permeability of the proximal tubule to water, this small osmotic pressure gradient is sufficient to cause water reabsorption. Also, as water flows from the lumen to the interstitium, it brings additional solute with it via solvent drag.

When an osmotic diuretic is present in the tubular fluid, its concentration increases progressively as a result of NaCl and water reabsorption by the nephron. With this increase in concentration, an osmotic gradient develops opposite to the normal gradient generated by the NaCl reabsorptive process. As a result, both NaCl (solvent drag component) and water reabsorption are reduced.

A portion of the Na^+ that is not reabsorbed by the proximal tubule is reabsorbed downstream by the thick ascending limb. Because this segment can significantly increase its reabsorption when challenged with a large delivered load, the degree of natriuresis seen with osmotic diuretics is less than expected based on the magnitude of proximal tubule reabsorption. Although Na^+ excretion rates as high as 60% of the filtered load have been observed in experimental situations, the natriuresis seen with osmotic diuretics is usually only about 10% of the filtered load.

Carbonic Anhydrase Inhibitors

Carbonic anhydrase inhibitors (e.g., acetazolamide) inhibit Na^+ reabsorption by their effect on carbonic anhydrase. This enzyme is abundant in the proximal tubule and therefore represents the major site of action of these diuretics. Carbonic anhydrase is also present in other cells along the nephron (e.g., intercalated cells of the collecting duct), and administration of carbonic anhydrase inhibitors affects the activity of the enzyme in these sites as well. However, the effects of these diuretics are almost entirely attributed to their inhibition of the enzyme in the proximal tubule.

As described in Chapter 8, carbonic anhydrase is critical for the reabsorption of HCO_3^- by the proximal tubule. In this segment, the enzyme is located within the cell and in the apical membrane. The intracellular enzyme facilitates the formation of H^+ and HCO_3^- from CO_2 and H_2O. HCO_3^- exits the cell across the basolateral membrane and returns to the blood, whereas H^+ is secreted into the tubular fluid in exchange for Na^+. In the tubular fluid, H^+ combines with the filtered HCO_3^- to form H_2CO_3. This is rapidly hydrolyzed to CO_2 and H_2O by the carbonic anhydrase located in the apical membrane, thus facilitating CO_2 and H_2O reabsorption. The activities of the apical membrane and intracellular enzymes are decreased by the carbonic anhydrase inhibitors, which significantly reduces the reabsorption of HCO_3^-. Because the process of H^+ secretion and thus HCO_3^- reabsorption by the proximal tubule cells is dependent upon Na^+ (Na^+-H^+ antiporter in the apical membrane), inhibition of

carbonic anhydrase also results in a decrease in Na^+ reabsorption.

Approximately one third of all proximal tubule Na^+ reabsorption is related to the process of HCO_3^- reabsorption. Inhibition of this process by the carbonic anhydrase inhibitors would therefore be expected to cause a large increase in Na^+ excretion (as much as 20% to 30% of the filtered load). However, this is not the case; Na^+ excretion rates of only 5% to 10% of the filtered load are observed with these diuretics. The reason for this is the same as that described for osmotic diuretics and relates to the ability of the thick ascending limb to increase its reabsorptive rate when delivery is increased.

Loop Diuretics

Loop diuretics (e.g., furosemide, bumetanide, and ethacrynic acid) are anions that enter the tubular lumen by glomerular filtration and via secretion by the organic anion secretory system of the proximal tubule. They inhibit Na^+ reabsorption by the thick ascending limb of Henle's loop by blocking the $1Na^+$-$2Cl^-$-$1K^+$ symporter located in the apical membrane of these cells (see Chapter 4). By this action, they not only inhibit Na^+ reabsorption but also disrupt the process of countercurrent multiplication. Because of this effect, loop diuretics impair the kidneys' ability to dilute and concentrate the urine. Dilution is impaired because solute (NaCl) reabsorption by the water-impermeable thick ascending limb of Henle's loop is inhibited. Because NaCl reabsorption by the medullary portion of the thick ascending limb is critical for the generation and maintenance of the medullary interstitial osmotic gradient, inhibition of transport by loop diuretics results in a decrease in this gradient. With a decrease in medullary interstitial osmolality, water reabsorption from the collecting duct is impaired, and the concentrating ability of the kidneys is reduced. Water reabsorption from the thin descending limb of Henle's loop is also impaired, which accounts in part for the increase in water excretion seen with loop diuretics.

Loop diuretics are the most potent diuretics available, increasing the excretion of Na^+ to 20% to 25% of the filtered load. This large natriuresis reflects the fact that the thick ascending limb normally reabsorbs approximately 20% to 25% of the filtered load of Na^+, and the downstream segments have a limited capacity to compensate for the increased delivered load of Na^+ received as a result of the diuretics actions.

Thiazide Diuretics

Thiazide diuretics (e.g., chlorothiazide and metolazone),* like the loop diuretics, are anions that gain access to the tubular lumen by filtration and secretion in the proximal tubule. They act to inhibit Na^+ reabsorption in the early portion of the distal tubule by blocking the NaCl symporter in the apical membrane of these cells (see Chapter 4). Because this portion of the nephron is impermeable to water, it is a site of urine dilution. Therefore, by inhibiting NaCl reabsorption, thiazides block urine dilution. Natriuresis with thiazide diuretics is 5% to 10% of the filtered load and is a direct reflection of the amount of Na^+ normally reabsorbed by the distal tubule.

K^+-Sparing Diuretics

The K^+-*sparing diuretics* act on the region of the nephron where K^+ secretion occurs (late portion of the distal tubule and cortical collecting duct). Because the amount of Na^+ reabsorbed by this region is small (2% to 3%), these diuretics do not produce significant natriuresis. As the name implies, their utility lies in their ability to inhibit K^+ secretion by this region of the nephron.

There are two classes of K^+-sparing diuretics:

one acts by antagonizing aldosterone's action on the collecting duct principal cell (e.g., spironolactone), while the other class blocks the entry of Na^+ into these same cells through the Na^+-selective channels in the apical membrane (e.g., amiloride and triamterene). These latter two diuretics are cations that enter the tubular lumen by glomerular filtration and secretion by the organic cation secretory system of the proximal tubule.

The reabsorption of Na^+ and the secretion of K^+ by the principal cell of the collecting duct are stimulated by aldosterone. Aldosterone acts by increasing the number of functional Na^+ and K^+ channels in the apical membrane and the levels of Na^+-K^+-ATPase in the basolateral membrane (see Chapters 6 and 7). By this action, Na^+ entry into the cell from the lumen is enhanced, as is its extrusion from the cell across the basolateral membrane. Similarly, the blood-to-lumen movement of K^+ is enhanced. In the presence of an aldosterone antagonist, these effects are reversed, and both Na^+ reabsorption and K^+ secretion are reduced.

The ability of the Na^+ channel blockers amiloride and triamterene to inhibit Na^+ reabsorption and K^+ secretion is similar to that of spironolactone, but the cellular mechanism is different (Figure 10-3). These drugs interact directly with the Na^+-selective channel in the apical membrane of the principal cell and block the entry of Na^+. With decreased Na^+ entry, there is decreased Na^+ extrusion across the basolateral membrane via Na^+-K^+-ATPase. This in turn reduces cellular K^+ uptake and ultimately its secretion into the tubular fluid. The blockade of the apical membrane Na^+ channels also alters the electrical profile across the luminal membrane, with the voltage across this membrane increasing in magnitude. Because of this voltage change, the electrochemical gradient for K^+ movement out of the cell is reduced. This membrane voltage effect also contributes to the inhibition of K^+ secretion.

*Metolazone is not of the same chemical class of drugs as the thiazides. However, because its site of action is the same, it is grouped with this class of diuretics.

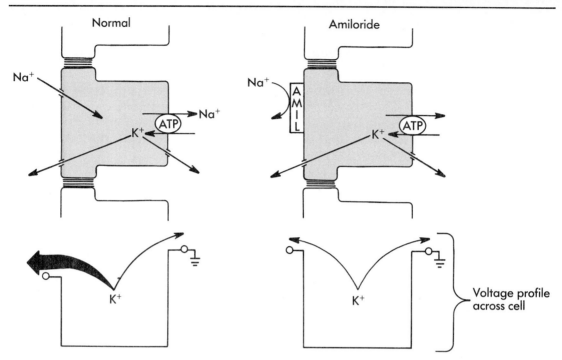

Figure 10-3 ■ Effect of the K⁺-sparing diuretic amiloride (Amil) on the electrical profile across the principal cell of the cortical collecting duct. By blocking the apical membrane Na⁺ channels, the voltage across this membrane is hyperpolarized. This in turn reduces the gradient for cell-to-lumen diffusion of K⁺. Also, decreased cell Na⁺ entry across the apical membrane reduces the activity of the Na⁺-K⁺-ATPase, and thereby K⁺ uptake into the cell across the basolateral membrane. Together, these effects inhibit K⁺ secretion.

■ EFFECT OF DIURETICS ON THE EXCRETION OF WATER AND OTHER SOLUTES

Through their effects on Na⁺ handling along the nephron, diuretics also influence the handling of water and other solutes. Table 10-1 summarizes the effects of the various diuretic agents on the handling of some of these solutes and the ability of the kidneys to excrete (C_{H_2O}) and conserve ($T^c_{H_2O}$) solute-free water.

Solute-Free Water

As discussed in Chapter 5, the ability of the kidneys to either excrete or reabsorb solute-free water depends on several factors. With regard to the action of diuretic agents, the factors of concern are:

1. The normal function of the nephron segments (particularly the thick ascending limb).
2. The delivery of adequate solute to Henle's loop.
3. The maintenance of a hyperosmotic medullary interstitium (reabsorption of solute-free water only).

The thick ascending limb of Henle's loop is the most important site for the separation of solute and water. As noted above, this separation not only dilutes the tubular fluid, but, by establishing a hyperosmotic medullary interstitium, allows for concentration of the urine as well. Inhibition of thick ascending limb reabsorption by loop diuretics therefore results in inhibition of both C_{H_2O} and $T^c_{H_2O}$.

Table 10-1 ■ Urinary excretion of water and some solutes with diuretics

Diuretic	Na+ excretion (%)*	K+ excretion	HCO₃⁻ excretion	Ca++ excretion	C_{H_2O}	$T^c_{H_2O}$
Osmotic diuretic	10	↑	↑	↑	↑	↑
Acetazolamide	5	↑	↑	↑	↑	↑
Bumetanide	25	↑	↓	↑	↓	↓
Ethacrynic acid	25	↑	↓	↑	↓	↓
Furosemide	25	↑	↓	↑	↓	↓
Chlorothiazide	8	↑	↓	↓	↓	Unchanged
Metolazone	8	↑	↓	↓	↓	Unchanged
Amiloride	2	↓	↑	Unchanged	Unchanged	Unchanged
Spironolactone	2	↓	↑	Unchanged	Unchanged	Unchanged
Triamterene	2	↓	↑	Unchanged	Unchanged	Unchanged

*Percent of filtered load excreted into urine

The early portion of the distal tubule is also a site of solute and water separation, and thus tubular fluid dilution. Accordingly, inhibition of transport by thiazide diuretics impairs dilution of the urine and thus reduces C_{H_2O}. Thiazide diuretics impair urine dilution to a lesser degree than do loop diuretics, reflecting the difference in NaCl reabsorptive capacity between the early portion of the distal tubule (5% to 10% of the filtered load) and the thick ascending limb (20% to 25% of the filtered load). In contrast to loop diuretics, thiazide diuretics do not significantly impair the ability of the kidneys to concentrate urine; this requires the maintenance of a normal medullary interstitial osmotic gradient. Because the cortex is the site of action of thiazide diuretics, their action at this site does not appreciably alter the medullary interstitial osmotic gradient. Consequently, urine concentrating ability and thus the generation of $T^c_{H_2O}$ are unaffected by thiazide diuretics.

The action of diuretics in the proximal tubule (osmotic diuretics and carbonic anhydrase inhibitors) results in an increase in the delivery of NaCl and water to Henle's loop. In view of the thick ascending limb's ability to increase its transport rate, there is an increase in the separation of solute and water with this increased delivery. As a result, these diuretic agents increase the ability of the kidneys to produce either C_{H_2O} or $T^c_{H_2O}$.

Although the late portion of the distal tubule and the collecting duct are able to dilute the luminal fluid in the absence of ADH, Na+ transport in these segments is not of sufficient magnitude to significantly contribute to the generation of C_{H_2O}. Consequently, the K+-sparing diuretics do not appreciably alter this parameter nor the kidneys' ability to generate $T^c_{H_2O}$.

K+ Handling

One of the major consequences of diuretic use (excluding K+-sparing diuretics) is increased excretion of K+. This can be of sufficient magnitude to result in hypokalemia. The basis for this diuretic-induced increase in renal K^+ excretion lies in the fact that, when a diuretic inhibits Na^+ and water reabsorption in segments upstream from the late portion of the distal tubule and cortical collecting duct (K^+ secretory site of the nephron), there is an increase in tubular fluid flow rate and the delivery of additional amounts of Na^+ to this nephron region. Both of these factors stimulate K^+ secretion at this site (see Chapter 7). In addition, by their action on Na^+ balance, diuretics decrease ECF volume. This in turn leads to increased secretion of aldosterone by the adrenal cortex (see Chapter 6), which acts at this site to stimulate K^+ secretion. The K^+-sparing diuretics prevent the increase in K^+ excretion caused by the other diuretics; therefore, they are usually given in combination with these other diuretics to prevent, or at least minimize, the development of hypokalemia.

HCO_3^- Handling

By inhibiting HCO_3^- reabsorption in the proximal tubule and thereby increasing HCO_3^- excretion, carbonic anhydrase inhibitors can result in the development of a metabolic acidosis. With this acidosis, the filtered load of HCO_3^- is reduced (i.e., the plasma $[HCO_3^-]$ is reduced). This results in less HCO_3^- available for reabsorption, which diminishes the effectiveness of carbonic anhydrase inhibitors.

Although only carbonic anhydrase inhibitors directly alter HCO_3^- handling by the nephron, all diuretics can secondarily affect systemic acid-base balance. Both loop diuretics and thiazides can induce a metabolic alkalosis, which is a consequence of the decrease in ECF volume that accompanies their use. With a decrease in ECF volume, Na^+ is more avidly reabsorbed in the proximal tubule (see Chapter 6). Because HCO_3^- is reabsorbed together with Na^+ in this segment, proximal tubule HCO_3^- reabsorption is increased. Additionally, the reduction in ef-

fective circulating volume stimulates aldosterone secretion by the adrenal cortex. As discussed in Chapter 8, aldosterone stimulates collecting duct H^+ secretion. Because proximal tubule HCO_3^- reabsorption is increased, virtually none of the filtered load of HCO_3^- reaches the collecting duct. Therefore, the increased H^+ secretion that occurs in the collecting duct results in the production of new HCO_3^- as the H^+ is excreted with non-HCO_3^- urinary buffers (e.g., NH_4^+ and T.A.). This new HCO_3^- is added to the plasma and produces a metabolic alkalosis.

By inhibiting Na^+ reabsorption in the late portion of the distal tubule and cortical collecting duct, K^+-sparing diuretics secondarily inhibit H^+ secretion and can lead to the development of a metabolic acidosis. H^+ secretion is facilitated by a lumen-negative transepithelial voltage. Normally, Na^+ reabsorption in these nephron segments results in the generation of such a voltage. By inhibiting Na^+ reabsorption and thus the negative luminal voltage, K^+-sparing diuretics reduce H^+ secretion. With reduced H^+ secretion, insufficient quantities of net acid are excreted, and a metabolic acidosis ensues.

Ca^{++}, Mg^{++}, and PO_4^{3-} Handling

With the exception of K^+-sparing diuretics, all of the diuretics can significantly alter Ca^{++} handling by the kidney. With inhibition of proximal tubule solute and water reabsorption (osmotic diuretics and carbonic anhydrase inhibitors), there is reduced reabsorption of Ca^{++} and thus increased excretion. The amount of Ca^{++} excreted is variable and generally less than that which is expected from inhibition of proximal tubule transport. This again reflects the ability of the downstream segments (particularly the thick ascending limb of Henle's loop) to increase reabsorption following an increased delivered load. The mechanism by which these diuretics inhibit proximal tubule Ca^{++} reabsorption is related to their ability to reduce solvent drag (see Chapter 9). With the use of carbonic anhydrase inhibitors, increased Ca^{++} excretion occurs in the setting of an alkaline urine (increased urinary $[HCO_3^-]$). Because Ca^{++} is less soluble in alkaline urine, the potential exists for the formation of Ca^{++}-containing renal stones.

Loop diuretics also increase Ca^{++} excretion, an action explained by the effect of these diuretic agents on the transepithelial voltage of the thick ascending limb of Henle's loop. Normally, the transepithelial voltage of this limb is oriented lumen-positive (see Chapter 4), providing a driving force for the movement of Ca^{++} from the lumen to blood through the paracellular pathway. When transport of NaCl by Henle's loop is blocked by loop diuretics, this lumen-positive voltage is abolished, and the driving force for Ca^{++} reabsorption is reduced. Normally, Henle's loop reabsorbs about 20% of the filtered load of Ca^{++} (see Chapter 9). Inhibition of Ca^{++} reabsorption by loop diuretics can therefore have a significant effect on overall Ca^{++} balance. For this reason, loop diuretics are frequently used to treat hypercalcemia. Despite this action of loop diuretics, hypercalcemia can occur with their long-term use. The mechanism responsible for this effect is related to the diuretic-induced decrease in ECF volume. When ECF volume is decreased, proximal tubule reabsorption is enhanced, which in turn increases Ca^{++} reabsorption at this site, and therefore decreases urinary Ca^{++} excretion.

Thiazide diuretics stimulate Ca^{++} reabsorption by the cells of the early portion of the distal tubule, and thus reduce its excretion. The early distal tubule normally reabsorbs 5% to 10% of the filtered load of Ca^{++} (see Chapter 9). The reabsorption of Ca^{++} at this site is an active transcellular process, although the specific mechanisms for this have not yet been defined. Nor has it been determined by what mechanism thiazide diuretics stimulate Ca^{++} reabsorption.

Because thiazides reduce urinary Ca^{++} excretion, they are sometimes used to lower the incidence of Ca^{++} stone formation in individuals who normally excrete high levels of Ca^{++} in their urine.

Because only small quantities of Ca^{++} are reabsorbed by the collecting duct, K^+-sparing diuretics do not have an appreciable effect on urinary Ca^{++} excretion.

In general, changes in the excretion of Mg^{++} with administration of diuretics parallel those described for Ca^{++}. There is, however, one important difference: thiazide diuretics cause a slight increase in Mg^{++} excretion, which is the opposite of their effect on Ca^{++} excretion.

The mechanisms by which the various diuretics affect Mg^{++} handling by the nephron are not fully understood. It is believed that diuretics acting in the proximal tubule inhibit Mg^{++} reabsorption by reducing solvent drag. Because the thick ascending limb reabsorbs the largest portion of the filtered load of Mg^{++} (see Chapter 9), administration of a loop diuretic can result in the excretion of large amounts of Mg^{++}. This effect, like that seen for Ca^{++}, is related to the loop diuretic-induced inhibition of the lumen-positive transepithelial voltage of the thick ascending limb of Henle's loop. This reduces passive Mg^{++} reabsorption via the paracellular pathways. Because the distal tubule and collecting duct have little capacity to reabsorb the increased delivered load of Mg^{++}, excretion is increased. As noted, thiazide diuretics slightly increase the excretion of Mg^{++}, although the mechanism for this effect is unknown. Finally, K^+-sparing diuretics do not appreciably alter Mg^{++} excretion.

With the exception of the K^+-sparing diuretics, all diuretics acutely increase PO_4^{3-} excretion. However, the cellular mechanisms for this effect are not completely understood. The effect is modified, however, with long-term diuretic therapy. With the decrease in ECF volume that accompanies long-term diuretic use, proximal tubule Na^+ reabsorption is stimulated. Because the proximal tubule reabsorbs the largest portion of the filtered load of PO_4^{3-}, and because this reabsorptive process is coupled with Na^+ (see Chapters 4 and 9), PO_4^{3-} excretion is reduced in this setting.

■ KEY WORDS AND CONCEPTS

- Natriuresis
- Steady-state balance
- Organic anion and organic cation secretory systems
- Osmotic diuretics
- Carbonic anhydrase inhibitors
- Loop diuretics
- Thiazide diuretics
- K^+-sparing diuretics

■ SELF-STUDY PROBLEMS

1. Diuretics are administered to two groups of individuals: Group 1 subjects are water-loaded and produce dilute urine, whereas Group 2 subjects are water-deprived and produce concentrated urine. After control urine and plasma samples are obtained, each individual receives one of three diuretics, and urine and plasma samples are again obtained. Calculate C_{H_2O} and $T^c_{H_2O}$. Based on the effect of the diuretics on these parameters, identify the class of diuretic administered.

Condition	P_{osm} (mOsm/kg H_2O)	U_{osm} (mOsm/kg H_2O)	$\dot{V}$ (ml/min)	C_{H_2O} (ml/min)	$T^c_{H_2O}$ (ml/min)
Water Diuresis					
Before diuretic A	285	70	10	_____	
After diuretic A	284	125	16	_____	
Before diuretic B	286	65	12	_____	
After diuretic B	286	200	19	_____	
Before diuretic C	284	70	11	_____	
After diuretic C	285	195	15	_____	
Antidiuresis					
Before diuretic A	288	1,200	0.6		_____
After diuretic A	289	450	12.0		_____
Before diuretic B	290	1,100	0.7		_____
After diuretic B	288	300	13.0		_____
Before diuretic C	287	1,200	0.7		_____
After diuretic C	290	355	10.0		_____

Diuretic A: _____

Diuretic B: _____

Diuretic C: _____

2. Patients with nephrogenic diabetes insipidus can obtain symptomatic relief from their polyuria with long-term use of a thiazide diuretic. What is the mechanism by which long-term thiazide therapy produces a decrease in urine volume in these patients?

3. An individual is begun on a thiazide diuretic as partial therapy for hypertension. Prior to therapy, plasma $[K^+]$ is 4.0 mEq/L. After several months of therapy, the individual's blood pressure is reduced and plasma $[K^+]$ is 3.0 mEq/L.

   a. By what mechanism could the diuretic lead to a decrease in blood pressure?

   b. By what mechanism did the plasma $[K^+]$ fall? What other classes of diuretics would produce this effect?

   c. What can be done to increase plasma $[K^+]$ to the level it was prior to beginning diuretic therapy?

4. The antibiotic penicillin is secreted into the urine by the organic anion secretory system of the proximal tubule. If an individual taking a thiazide diuretic for hypertension develops an infection requiring penicillin, what effect, if any, could this have on the action of the diuretic?

Additional Reading

■ GENERAL

Brenner BM and Rector FC Jr (editors): The kidney, ed 4, Philadelphia, 1991, WB Saunders Co. *(A two-volume, comprehensive text on the kidney. Includes sections on normal physiology, pathophysiology, and clinical nephrology. Each chapter is written by experts in the field and includes an extensive list of references.)*

Rose BD: Clinical physiology of acid-base and electrolyte disorders, ed 3, New York, 1989, McGraw-Hill Inc. *(Clearly written book that discusses fluid and electrolyte disorders from basic physiological principles.)*

Seldin DW and Giebisch G (editors): The kidney: physiology and pathophysiology, ed 2, New York, 1992, Raven Press. *(A two-volume, comprehensive text on the kidney, similar in many ways to the Brenner and Rector text. Includes sections on normal physiology, pathophysiology, and clinical nephrology. Each chapter is written by experts in the field and includes an extensive list of references.)*

Seldin DW and Giebisch G (editors): The regulation of sodium and chloride balance, New York, 1990, Raven Press. *(Concise review of Na⁺ handling by the kidney and the regulation of Na⁺ balance. Includes both normal physiology and pathophysiology.)*

Seldin DW and Giebisch G (editors): The regulation of acid-base balance, New York, 1990, Raven Press. *(Concise review of all aspects of acid-base homeostasis, including both renal and respiratory control. Basic physiology and pathophysiology are discussed.)*

Seldin DW and Giebisch G (editors): The regulation of potassium balance, New York, 1989, Raven Press. *(Concise review of all aspects of K⁺ homeostasis. Basic physiology and pathophysiology are discussed.)*

■ CHAPTER 1

Badr K and Ichikawa I: Physical and biological properties of body fluid electrolytes. In Ichikawa (editor): Pediatric textbook of fluids and electrolytes, Baltimore, 1990, Williams & Wilkins. *(Reviews the basic physicochemical properties of electrolyte solutions.)*

Fanestil DD: Compartmentation of body water. In Maxwell MH, Kleeman CR, and Narins RG (editors): Clinical disorders of fluid and electrolyte metabolism, ed 4, New York, 1987, McGraw-Hill Inc. *(Reviews techniques for measuring the volumes of the body fluid compartments. Regulation of cell volume under normal and pathophysiological conditions is also considered.)*

Rose BD: Clinical physiology of acid-base and electrolyte disorders, ed 3, New York, 1989, McGraw-Hill Inc. *(Chapter 1 discusses the basic principles of ions in solution. The volumes and compositions of the various body fluid compartments are also described.)*

Yoshioka T, Iitaka K, and Ichikawa I: Body fluid compartments. In Ichikawa I (editor): Pediatric textbook of fluids and electrolytes, Baltimore, 1990, Williams & Wilkins. *(Describes the volumes and compositions of the various body fluid compartments.)*

■ CHAPTER 2

Bradley WE: Physiology of the urinary bladder. In Walsh PC et al (editors): Cambell's urology, ed 5, Philadelphia, 1986, WB Saunders Co. *(A very thorough treatise on the physiology of the lower urinary tract.)*

Kriz W and Bankir L: A standard nomenclature for structures of the kidney, Am J Physiol 254: F1, 1988. *(A complete review of renal nomenclature providing most synonyms for each structure. Does not, however, contain any references.)*

Kriz W and Kaissling B: Structural organization of the mammalian kidney. In Seldin DW and Giebisch G (editors): The kidney: physiology and pathophysiology, ed 2, New York, 1992, Raven Press. *(A complete and detailed review of renal structure with numerous references and superb electron micrographs.)*

Tanagho EA: Anatomy of the lower urinary tract. In Walsh PC et al (editors): Cambell's urology, ed 5, Philadelphia, 1986, WB Saunders Co. *(A very thorough treatise on the anatomy of the lower urinary tract.)*

Tanagho EA: Anatomy of the geniturinary tract. In Tanagho EA and McAnich JW (editors): Smith's general urology, ed 12, Norwalk, 1988, Appleton & Lange. *(One of the standard texts on urology for medical students and urology residents. Very concise with numerous illustrations.)*

Tisher CC and Madsen KM: Anatomy of the kidney. In Brenner BM and Rector FC Jr (editors): The kidney, ed 4, Philadelphia, 1991, WB Saunders Co. *(A complete and detailed review of renal structure and ultrastructure. Superb electron micrographs.)*

■ CHAPTER 3

Baylis C and Blantz RC: Glomerular hemodynamics, News in Physiol Sci 1: 86, 1986. *(A brief overview of glomerular hemodynamics.)*

Gottschalk CW (editor): Renal and electrolyte physiology section: Tubuloglomerular feedback mechanisms, Annu Rev Physiol 49: 249, 1987. *(This volume contains three reviews on tubuloglomerular feedback.)*

Dworkin LD and Brenner BM: The biophysical basis of glomerular filtration. In Seldin DW and Giebisch G (editors): The kidney: physiology and pathophysiology, ed 2, New York, 1992, Raven Press. *(A complete review of the biophysics of glomerular filtration.)*

Dworkin LD and Brenner BM: The renal circulations. In Brenner BM and Rector FC Jr (editors): The kidney, ed 4, Philadelphia, 1991, WB Saunders Co. *(Superb illustrations of the renal circulatory system. A very detailed review of the anatomy of the vasculature.)*

Kassier JP and Harrington JT: Laboratory evaluation of renal function. In Schrier RW and Gottschalk CW (editors): Diseases of the kidney, ed 4, Boston, 1988, Little, Brown & Co Inc. *(Describes the general approach for the clinical evaluation of renal function. The use of creatinine clearance for the measurement of glomerular filtration rate is discussed.)*

Koushanpour E and Kriz W: Renal physiology, ed 2, Berlin, 1986, Springer-Verlag, New York Inc. *(Chapter 7 describes the use of inulin and creatinine to measure the glomerular filtration rate, and PAH to measure renal plasma flow.)*

Maddox DA and Brenner BM: Glomerular ultrafiltration. In Brenner BM and Rector FC Jr (editors): The kidney, ed 4, Philadelphia, 1991, WB Saunders Co. *(An advanced review of glomerular ultrafiltration with complete presentations on hormonal regulation of GFR and RBF, autoregulation of GFR, and tubuloglomerular feedback.)*

Schuster VL and Seldin DW: Renal clearance. In Seldin DW and Giebisch G (editors): The kidney: physiology and pathophysiology, ed 2, New York, 1992, Raven Press. *(An in-depth review of the concept of renal clearance as applied to the normal and diseased kidney.)*

Ulfendahl H and Wolgast M: Renal circulation and lymphatics. In Seldin DW and Giebisch G (editors): The kidney: physiology and pathophysiology, ed 2, New York, 1992, Raven Press. *(A review of the functional aspects of renal circulation, including autoregulation of RBF and the pathophysiology of renal circulation.)*

■ CHAPTER 4

Berry CA and Rector FC Jr: Renal transport of glucose, amino acids, sodium, chloride, and water. In Brenner BM and Rector FC Jr (editors): The kidney, ed 4, Philadelphia, 1991, WB Saunders Co. *(A complete and up-to-date review of solute transport along the nephron.)*

Byrne JH and Schultz SG: An introduction to membrane transport and bioelectricity, New York, 1988, Raven Press. *(A clearly written book reviewing the principles of membrane transport and bioelectricity, without the use of complex and complicated mathematics. Intended for medical students and beginning graduate students.)*

Giebisch G and Boulpaep EL (editors): Symposium on cotransport mechanisms in renal tubules, Kidney Int 36: 333, 1989. *(An up-to-date review of antiport and symport transport mechanisms and organic anion transport mechanisms in the nephron.)*

■ CHAPTER 5

Gross P and Ritz E (editors): Water metabolism, Kidney Int Suppl 21, 1987. *(This entire supplement reviews the synthesis, secretion, and actions of ADH; the urine concentrating and diluting processes; and clinical disorders of water balance.)*

Hays RM: Cell biology of vasopressin. In Brenner BM and Rector FC Jr (editors): The kidney, ed 4, Philadelphia, 1991, WB Saunders Co. *(A detailed and up-to-date review of the actions of ADH on its target cells. Emphasis is placed on the membrane and biochemical events associated with ADH action.)*

Knepper MA and Rector FC Jr: Urinary concentration and dilution. In Brenner BM and Rector FC Jr (editors): The kidney, ed 4, Philadelphia, 1991, WB Saunders Co. *(A detailed and up-to-date review of the urine concentration and dilution processes. Summarizes current research findings and identifies unresolved questions.)*

Robertson GL and Berl T: Pathophysiology of water metabolism. In Brenner BM and Rector FC Jr (editors): The kidney, ed 4, Philadelphia, 1991, WB Saunders Co. *(Reviews the control of ADH secretion and the thirst system. Also included is a discussion of disorders of water balance.)*

A *first-rate reference for the advanced student or clinician.)*

■ CHAPTER 6

Brenner BM et al: Diverse biological actions of atrial natriuretic peptide, Physiol Rev 70: 665, 1990. *(A comprehensive review of the actions of ANP. Considerable detail is presented on the cellular mechanisms of action on the kidneys and other organs.)*

Little RC and Ginsburg JM: The physiological basis for clinical edema, Arch Intern Med 144: 1661, 1984. *(A brief review of the dynamics of capillary fluid exchange and how alterations in the Starling forces can result in the accumulation of excess fluid in the interstitial space.)*

Marver D (editor): Corticosteroids and the kidney, Semin Nephrol 10:311, 1990. *(This entire issue reviews virtually all aspects of the actions of aldosterone on the kidney.)*

Moe GW, Legault L, and Skorecki KL: Control of extracellular fluid volume and pathophysiology of edema formation. In Brenner BM and Rector FC Jr (editors): The kidney, ed 4, Philadelphia, 1991, WB Saunders Co. *(A complete and up-to-date review of the control of renal Na+ handling and its relationship to the volume of the extracellular fluid compartment.)*

Sealey JE and Laragh JH: The integrated regulation of electrolyte balance and blood pressure by the renin system. In Seldin DW and Giebisch G (editors): The regulation of sodium and chloride balance, New York, 1990, Raven Press. *(A review of the renin-angiotensin-aldosterone system. Included are sections on the control of renin secretion, the actions of angiotensin II and aldosterone on the kidney, and interactions with ANP.)*

■ CHAPTER 7

Giebisch G, Malnic G, and Berliner RW: Renal transport and control of potassium excretion. In Brenner BM and Rector FC Jr (editors): The kidney, ed 4, Philadelphia, 1991, WB Saunders Co. *(A detailed review of the cellular mechanisms of potassium transport and the factors and hormones regulating urinary potassium excretion.)*

Stanton BA and Giebisch G: Renal potassium transport. In Windhager EE (editor): Handbook of physiology: renal physiology, ed 2, New York, 1992, Oxford University Press Inc. *(A detailed review of potassium homeostasis.)*

Seldin DW and Giebisch G (editors): The regulation of potassium balance, New York, 1989, Raven Press. *(14 Chapters on all aspects of K+ homeostasis, 7 chapters on normal K+ metabolism, and 7 on abnormal K+ metabolism.)*

■ CHAPTER 8

Alpern RJ, Stone DK, Rector FC Jr: Renal acidification mechanisms. In Brenner BM and Rector FC Jr (editors): The kidney, ed 4, Philadelphia, 1991, WB Saunders Co. *(A comprehensive review of renal H^+, HCO_3^-, and NH_4^+ handling.)*

Cogan MG and Rector FC Jr: Acid-base disorders. In Brenner BM and Rector FC Jr (editors): The kidney, ed 4, Philadelphia, 1991, WB Saunders Co. *(Reviews the etiology and pathophysiology of metabolic acidosis and alkalosis. The general approach to diagnosis of acid-base disorders is also provided.)*

DuBose TD Jr: Reclamation of filtered bicarbonate, Kidney Int 38: 584, 1990. *(A brief review of the mechanisms of HCO_3^- reabsorption along the nephron.)*

Gluck SL: Cellular and molecular aspects of renal H^+ transport, Hosp Pract 24: 149, 1989. *(A review of the cellular and molecular mechanisms of H^+ secretion by the various segments of the nephron.)*

Knepper MA, Packer R, and Good DW: Ammonia transport in the kidney, Physiol Rev 69: 179, 1989. *(A comprehensive, in-depth review of the production and excretion of NH_4^+ by the kidney and the role it plays in net acid excretion.)*

Seldin DW and Giebisch G (editors): The regulation of acid-base balance, New York, 1990, Raven Press. *(This book covers all aspects of whole body acid-base balance, including the processes of buffering and respiratory compensation. The major emphasis is on the role of the kidney.)*

Valtin H and Gennari FJ: Acid-base disorders: basic concepts and clinical management, Boston, 1987, Little, Brown & Co Inc. *(A concise book on acid-base balance, with a focus on the major concepts and principles.)*

■ CHAPTER 9

Berndt T and Knox FG: Renal regulation of phosphate excretion. In Seldin DW and Giebisch G (editors): The kidney: physiology and pathophysiology, ed 2, New York, 1992, Raven Press. *(A thorough review of PO_4^{3-} excretion by the kidneys.)*

Suki WN and Rouse D: Renal transport of calcium, magnesium. In Brenner BM and Rector FC Jr (editors): The kidney, ed 4, Philadelphia, 1991, WB Saunders Co. *(A detailed review of renal and extrarenal mechanisms of Ca^{++}, Mg^{++}, and PO_4^{3-} homeostatic mechanisms.)*

Friedman PA: Renal calcium transport: sites and insights, News in Physiol Sci 3: 17, 1988. *(A brief overview of calcium transport along the nephron and its regulation.)*

■ CHAPTER 10

Breyer J and Jacobson HR: Molecular mechanisms of diuretic agents, Annu Rev Med 41: 265, 1990. *(Focuses on the transport mechanisms that are important for understanding the action of diuretics.)*

Friedman PA: Biochemistry and pharmacology of diuretics, Semin Nephrol 8: 198, 1988. *(Reviews the chemical nature and actions of the various classes of diuretic agents.)*

Rose BD: Nephrology forum: diuretics, Kidney Int 39: 336, 1991. *(A concise and complete review of the actions and uses of diuretics.)*

Thier SO: Diuretic mechanisms as a guide to therapy, Hosp Pract 22: 81, 1987. *(This review provides the mechanistic basis for the clinical use of the various classes of diuretics.)*

A Answers to Self-Study Problems

■ **CHAPTER 1**

1. a. Total body water (TBW) is calculated from the volume of distribution of tritiated water (THO). The amount of THO in the body is calculated as:

$$\begin{aligned} \text{Amount infused} &- \text{amount excreted} \\ &= \text{amount THO in body} \\ 5 \times 10^6 \text{ cpm} &- 2 \times 10^5 \text{ cpm} \\ &= 4.8 \times 10^6 \text{ cpm} \end{aligned}$$

The volume of distribution is then calculated as:

$$\begin{aligned} \text{Volume of distribution (TBW)} &= \frac{\text{amount THO}}{[\text{THO}]} \\ &= \frac{4.8 \times 10^6 \text{ cpm}}{10^5 \text{ cpm/L}} \\ &= 48 \text{ L} \end{aligned}$$

b. ECF volume is calculated from the volume of distribution of inulin, which is a marker for this compartment. The same approach, as outlined above for the calculation of TBW, is used.

$$\text{ECF volume} = \frac{20 \text{ g} - 12 \text{ g}}{0.5 \text{ g/L}} = 16 \text{ L}$$

c. There is no marker for the volume of the ICF. It is calculated from the difference between the TBW and ECF volume.

$$\text{ICF volume} = 48 \text{ L} - 16 \text{ L} = 32 \text{ L}$$

2. Na^+, with its anions Cl^- and HCO_3^-, constitutes the majority of particles in the ECF and is therefore the major determinant of plasma osmolality. Consequently, plasma osmolality can be estimated by simply doubling plasma $[Na^+]$. Thus, the estimated plasma osmolality in this individual is:

$$P_{osm} = 2(130) = 260 \text{ mOsm/kg } H_2O$$

This value is well below the normal range of 280 to 290 mOsm/kg H_2O and will result in movement of water from the ECF into cells. Because ions move freely across the capillary endothelium, the $[Na^+]$ (and osmolality) in the plasma and interstitial fluid will be the same. Therefore, there will be no effect on water movement across the capillary endothelium.

3. The initial volumes of the body fluid compartments and the osmoles in these compartments are calculated as (osmolality is estimated as $2 \times [Na^+]$):

Initial total body water = 0.6 × (60 kg) = 36 L
Initial ICF volume = 0.4 × (60 kg) = 24 L
Initial ECF volume = 0.2 × (60 kg) = 12 L
Initial total body osmoles = (total body water)(body fluid osmolality)
= (36 L)(280 mOsm/kg H_2O) = 10,080 mOsm
Initial ICF osmoles = (ICF volume)(body fluid osmolality)
= (24 L)(280 mOsm/kg H_2O) = 6,720 mOsm
Initial ECF osmoles = total body osmoles − ICF osmoles
= 10,080 mOsm − 6,720 mOsm = 3,360 mOsm

4 kg of body weight is lost. It is assumed that this entire weight reduction reflects fluids lost through vomiting and diarrhea. Thus, 4 L of fluid is lost. Because plasma [Na^+] is unchanged, a proportional amount of solute is also lost (isotonic loss of fluid). There will be no fluid shifts between the ECF and ICF, due to the absence of an osmotic gradient between these compartments. Thus, the ECF loses 4 L of volume and 4 × 140 = 560 mOsm of solute.

New total body water = 36 L − 4 L = 32 L
New ICF volume = 24 L (unchanged)
New ECF volume = 12 L − 4 L = 8 L
New total body osmoles = 10,080 mOsm − 560 mOsm = 9,520 mOsm
New ICF osmoles = 6,720 mOsm (unchanged)
New ECF osmoles = 3,360 mOsm − 560 mOsm = 2,800 mOsm

4. The initial volumes of the body fluid compartments and the osmoles in these compartments are calculated as for problem #3:

Initial total body water = 0.6 × (50 kg) = 30 L
Initial ICF volume = 0.4 × (50 kg) = 20 L
Initial ECF volume = 0.2 × (50 kg) = 10 L
Initial total body osmoles = (total body water)(body fluid osmolality)
= (30 L)(290 mOsm/kg H_2O) = 8,700 mOsm
Initial ICF osmoles = (ICF volume)(body fluid osmolality)
= (20 L)(290 mOsm/kg H_2O) = 5,800 mOsm
Initial ECF osmoles = total body osmoles − ICF osmoles
= 8,700 mOsm − 5,800 mOsm = 2,900 mOsm

To determine the effect of mannitol, the total amount infused must first be calculated. At 5 g/kg, a total of 250 g was infused (1.374 moles of mannitol). Because mannitol is a single particle in solution, this adds 1,374 mOsm to the ECF. The mannitol will raise ECF osmolality and result in the shift of fluid from the ICF into the ECF.

New total body water $\quad= 30$ L (unchanged)

New total body osmoles $= 8{,}700$ mOsm $+ 1{,}374$ mOsm $= 10{,}074$ mOsm

New ICF osmoles $\quad\quad= 5{,}800$ mOsm (unchanged)

New ECF osmoles $\quad\quad= 2{,}900$ mOsm $+ 1{,}374$ mOsm $= 4{,}274$ mOsm

$$\text{New plasma osmolality} = \frac{\text{new total osmoles}}{\text{total body water}}$$

$$= \frac{10{,}074 \text{ mOsm}}{30 \text{ L}} = 336 \text{ mOsm/kg } H_2O$$

$$\text{New ICF volume} = \frac{\text{ICF osmoles}}{\text{New } P_{osm}} = \frac{5{,}800 \text{ mOsm}}{336 \text{ mOsm/kg } H_2O} = 17.3 \text{ L}$$

$$\text{New ECF volume} = \text{total body water} - \text{ICF volume}$$

$$= 30 \text{ L} - 17.3 = 12.7 \text{ L}$$

Because mannitol increases the osmolality of the ECF, 2.7 L of fluid shifts from the ICF into the ECF. To calculate the new plasma $[Na^+]$, it is assumed that the amount of Na^+ in the ECF is unchanged after mannitol infusion. Originally, there were 2,900 mOsm due to Na^+ ($2 \times [Na^+] \times$ ECF volume) in the ECF. Because the Na^+ osmoles are unchanged but now present in a larger volume, the new plasma $[Na^+]$ is calculated as:

$$\text{New plasma } Na^+ \text{ osmoles} = \frac{2{,}900 \text{ mOsm due to } Na^+}{12.7 \text{ L}}$$

$$= 228 \text{ mOsm/L}$$

$$\text{New plasma } [Na^+] = \frac{Na^+ \text{ osmoles}}{2} = \frac{228 \text{ mOsm}}{2}$$

$$= 114 \text{ mEq/L}$$

5. Both individuals have lost water and solute from the body. Individual A lost 1 L of water and 1,200 mOsm of solute, while individual B lost 3 L of water and 900 mOsm of solute. Both have the same initial total body water (0.6×70 kg $= 42$ L) and total body osmoles ($290 \text{ mOsm/kg } H_2O \times 42 \text{ L} = 12{,}180$ mOsm). Their new P_{osm} values are calculated as:

$$P_{osm} (A) = \frac{12{,}180 \text{ mOsm} - 1{,}200 \text{ mOsm}}{42 \text{ L} - 1 \text{ L}}$$

$$= 268 \text{ mOsm/kg } H_2O$$

$$P_{osm} (B) = \frac{12{,}180 \text{ mOsm} - 900 \text{ mOsm}}{42 \text{ L} - 3 \text{ L}}$$

$$= 289 \text{ mOsm/kg } H_2O$$

■ CHAPTER 2

1. The five major segments of the nephron are the glomerulus, proximal tubule, Henle's loop, distal tubule, and collecting duct. The renal artery enters the kidney alongside the ureter and divides into the interlobular artery, the arcuate artery, the interlobar artery, and the afferent arteriole, which divides to form the glomerular capillaries. The glomerular capillaries coalesce to form the efferent arteriole, which leads into a second capillary network called the peritubular capillaries. Blood from the peritubular capillaries drains into the interlobular vein, arcuate vein, interlobar vein, and renal vein, which leaves the kidney alongside the ureter.

2. The glomerular capillaries have a fenestrated endothelium that prevents the filtration of cells. The endothelial cells are surrounded by a basement membrane composed of three layers (lamina rara interna, lamina densa, and lamina rara externa). The basement membrane is an important filtration barrier to plasma proteins. Filtration slits of the podocytes, which encircle the glomerular capillaries, are also a filtration barrier to proteins.

3. Structures that compose the juxtaglomerular apparatus include the macula densa of the thick ascending limb, extraglomerular mesangial cells, and the renin-producing cells of the afferent and efferent arterioles. The juxtaglomerular apparatus is one component of a feedback mechanism that regulates renal blood flow and glomerular filtration rate. Details of this mechanism are provided in Chapter 3.

4. Micturition is the process of emptying the urinary bladder. Filling of the bladder stretches the wall, which activates sensory nerves. These nerves send impulses from the bladder to the spinal cord via the pelvic nerves. Stretch stimulates the parasympathetic nerves, which cause intense contraction of the detrusor. This contraction, coupled with the voluntary relaxation of the external sphincter, allows urine to flow through the external meatus. Voluntary elimination of urine requires intact parasympathetic nerves and conscious control of the external sphincter.

■ CHAPTER 3

1. *Before pflorizin*
   Plasma [inulin]: 1 mg/ml
   Plasma [glucose]: 1 mg/ml
   Inulin excretion rate: 100 mg/min
   Glucose excretion rate: 0 mg/min
   Inulin clearance: ___100___ ml/min
   Glucose clearance: ___0___ ml/min

   After pflorizin
   Plasma [inulin]: 1 mg/ml
   Plasma [glucose]: 1 mg/ml
   Inulin excretion rate: 100 mg/min
   Glucose excretion rate: ___100___ mg/min
   Inulin clearance: ___100___ ml/min
   Glucose clearance: ___100___ ml/min

   Prior to pflorizin treatment, the filtered load of glucose (GFR $\times$ P_G) is 100 mg/min (GFR calculated from inulin clearance). This is below the T_m for glucose, and all of the glucose is reabsorbed, with none excreted. Thus, the clearance of glucose is zero. After pflorizin, the filtered load is unchanged, but there is no glucose reabsorption. Therefore, all of the glucose that is filtered is excreted, and the clearance of glucose equals that of inulin.

2. This problem makes use of the relationship:

   Excretion rate = filtered load − reabsorption rate + secretion rate
   $$U_x \times \dot{V} = (GFR \times P_x) - R + S$$

   Inulin: The clearance of inulin provides a measure of the GFR:

   $$GFR = \frac{U_{in} \times \dot{V}}{P_{in}}$$

   see table below

Substance	Urine [x] (mg/ml)	Plasma [x] (mg/ml)	$U_x \times \dot{V}$ (mg/min)	Clearance (ml/min)	Filtered load (mg/min)	Transport rate (mg/min)
Inulin	5.5	0.025	2.75	110.0	2.75	0
A	0.8	0.040	0.40	10.0	4.40	4.0 Reab.
B	7.5	0.068	3.75	55.1	3.74	≈0
C	11.0	0.010	5.50	550.0	1.10	4.4 Secrt.
D	10.0	0.060	5.0	83.3	1.65	3.4 Secrt.

a. This substance is freely filtered and almost entirely reabsorbed.

b. This substance is 50% bound to plasma protein. The total plasma [x] is used to calculate clearance, but only the free [x] is used to calculate the filtered load. Because the filtered load equals the excretion rate, there is no tubular transport.

c. This substance is freely filtered and also secreted.

d. This substance is 75% bound to plasma protein. Because the filtered load is less than the excretion rate, the substance is secreted.

Note: If it was not known that substances B and D were bound to plasma protein, examination of their clearances would have led to the erroneous conclusion that both were reabsorbed by the nephron.

3. a. Although red cells can appear in the urine as a result of damage to the glomerular filtration barrier, they can also appear in the urine for other reasons. For example, they can appear in the urine as a result of bleeding in any part of the lower urinary tract. Such bleeding occurs with kidney stones and occasionally from a bacterial infection of the lower urinary tract that causes bleeding. In women, urine can also contain menstrual blood.

b. Because glucose is filtered and completely reabsorbed by the proximal tubule, it is not normally found in the urine. Its presence in the urine indicates an elevated plasma glucose level, such that the filtered load (i.e., $GFR \times P_{glucose}$) is greater than the T_m for glucose reabsorption by the proximal tubule, or an abnormality in glucose transport. Since glucose is freely filtered by the normal glomerulus, damage to the ultrafiltration barrier would not increase its filtration.

c. Na^+ normally appears in the urine of healthy individuals. Like glucose, Na^+ is freely filtered by the normal glomerulus. Therefore, damage to the filtration barrier does not increase the rate of Na^+ excretion.

d. This is the correct answer. Normally, the urine contains essentially no protein, as the glomerulus prevents the filtration of plasma proteins. However, when damaged, large amounts of plasma proteins can be filtered. If the amount filtered overwhelms the reabsorptive capacity of the proximal tubule, protein appears in the urine (proteinuria).

4. The graph in the left column indicates the Starling forces along the glomerulus and how they change as filtration occurs. The Starling forces in glomerular and muscle capillaries are similar, except that the hydrostatic pressure in muscle capillaries decreases more rapidly along the length of the capillaries.

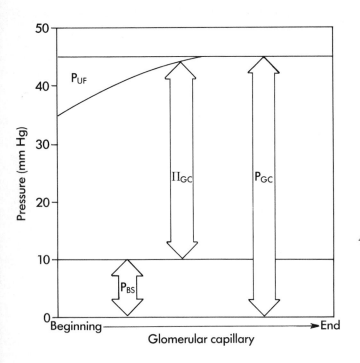

5. If plasma flow rate increases, more filtrate must be formed before the capillary oncotic pressure rises enough to stop filtration (i.e., $P_{UF} = 0$). Thus, at any point along a capillary, plasma oncotic pressure will be lower. Accordingly, the Starling forces across the glomerular capillary will be higher, and GFR will increase as flow increases.

6. The equation for blood flow through an organ is $Q = \Delta P/R$. Sympathetic agonists, angiotensin II, and prostaglandins change blood flow by altering the resistance (R). Sympathetic agonists and angiotensin II increase R and thereby decrease RBF, whereas prostaglandins decrease R and thereby increase RBF.

■ CHAPTER 4

1. The glomeruli filter 25,200 mEq of Na^+ and 18,000 mEq of Cl^- each day, with over 99% reabsorbed by the nephrons and only <1% appearing in the urine. Although Na^+ and Cl^- uptake into cells across the apical membrane and NaCl reabsorption across the paracellular pathway are passive processes (i.e., do not require the direct input of ATP), they ultimately depend on the operation of Na^+-K^+-ATPase. Accordingly, reabsorption of NaCl requires a considerable quantity of ATP. The synthesis of ATP by kidney cells requires large amounts of oxygen and thus a high blood flow.

2. There is really no such thing as "normal" or "average" urine composition, because of the variability in the volume excreted. Consider the table below.

Urine was collected on three different days from a subject who ate a constant diet but ingested different amounts of water each day. Although the amount of each solute excreted was similar on each day, the concentration of each solute in the urine was very different. This question illustrates that it is the amount of a solute excreted (or rate) that is important, not the concentration of the solute in the urine.

3. Passive transport always occurs down an electrochemical gradient. Diffusion of a solute through the lipid bilayer of the plasma membrane occurs passively. The text lists various types of transport proteins that mediate the passive movement of solutes across

	Urine Flow Rate		
	0.5 L/day	1.0 L/day	2.0 L/day
Na^+, mEq/L	300	150	75
K^+, mEq/L	200	100	50
Cl^-, mEq/L	300	150	75
HCO_3^-, mEq/L	≈4	≈2	≈1
Ca^{++}, mEq/L	20	10	5
NH_4^+, mEq/L	100	50	25
Creatinine, mg/L	2,000	1,000	500
Glucose, mmol/L	1.0	0.5	0.25
Urea, mmol/L	600	300	150
pH	5.0 . . . . to 7.0		
Osmolality, mOsm/kg H_2O	1,600	800	400

Modified from Valtin HV: Renal function, ed 2, Boston, 1983, Little, Brown & Co Inc. (pg. 298) and lab values from DMS (1989).

a membrane. With coupled transporters (antiport and symport), the movement of one molecule down its electrochemical gradient can drive uphill movement of the coupled molecule. When this occurs, the uphill movement is termed *secondary active* transport, because the transporter is not coupled directly to the hydrolysis of ATP. Active transport occurs against an electrochemical gradient and requires the direct input of energy (i.e., ATP). Some authors refer to such transport as *primary active* to emphasize the direct coupling to ATP. The text also lists some mechanisms of active transport.

4. Because Na^+-K^+-ATPase is ultimately responsible for the reabsorption and secretion of all solutes (except some H^+) and water by the nephron, complete inhibition of this transport protein blocks virtually all solute and water transport (both cellular and paracellular). Therefore, in this hypothetical example, each day the kidneys would excrete 180 L of fluid that would be similar in composition to the glomerular ultrafiltrate.

5. In the first phase of proximal reabsorption, Na^+ enters the cell across the apical membrane by several symport and antiport mechanisms (e.g., Na^+-glucose symport, Na^+-amino acid symport, and Na^+-H^+ antiport). Na^+ exit from the cell into the blood occurs by Na^+-K^+-ATPase. Therefore, Na^+ is reabsorbed across the cell with glucose, amino acids, and HCO_3^-. When tubular fluid reaches the second half of the proximal tubule, the concentrations of glucose, amino acids, and HCO_3^- are greatly reduced. As a result, the tubular fluid is primarily NaCl at this point. In the second phase of proximal tubule reabsorption, NaCl uptake across the apical membrane occurs by the parallel operation of Na^+-H^+ and Cl^--$Base^-$ antiporters. Na^+ efflux from the cell occurs via Na^+-K^+-ATPase, and Cl^- exits via Cl^- channels and KCl symport. Paracellular NaCl reabsorption also occurs.

Paracellular Cl^- reabsorption in the second half of the proximal tubule is driven by the Cl^- concentration gradient across the proximal tubule. This develops because relatively little Cl^- is reabsorbed in the first half of the proximal tubule (i.e., Na^+ is reabsorbed with other solutes). Cl^- diffusion across the tight junctions renders the transepithelial voltage lumen-positive, which in turn provides a driving force for the passive paracellular diffusion of Na^+. The transport of solutes (NaCl) across the cellular and paracellular pathways increases the osmolality of the interstitial fluid by ≈ 3 mOsm/kg H_2O, which establishes a driving force for water reabsorption across the proximal tubule. Some solutes are reabsorbed with this water by the process of solvent drag. Starling forces across the wall of the peritubular capillary are important for the uptake of this interstitial fluid and can regulate the rate of solute and water back-flux across the tight junctions, thereby modulating net solute and water reabsorption.

6. NaCl is reabsorbed across the thick ascending limb by two mechanisms: First, transcellular transport involves Na^+ and Cl^- entry into the cell across the apical membrane via the $1Na^+,2Cl^-,1K^+$ symporter (some additional Na^+ is reabsorbed by the apical membrane Na^+-H^+ antiporter) and exit across the basolateral membrane via Na^+-K^+-ATPase (for Na^+) and a KCl symporter and Cl^- channel (for Cl^-). Second, Na^+ is also reabsorbed across the paracellular pathway due to the lumen-positive transepithelial voltage. Furosemide would have no effect on water reabsorption, because this segment of the nephron is relatively impermeable to water, and water is not reabsorbed even when NaCl reabsorptive rates are high.

7. Glomerulotubular balance describes the phenomenon whereby an increase in the filtered load of water and NaCl is accompanied

by a parallel increase in NaCl and water reabsorption by the proximal tubule. If a constant amount of NaCl and water was reabsorbed by the proximal tubule, increases in GFR and the filtered load of NaCl and water would result in increased delivery to more distal segments. If these segments were not able to reabsorb the excess NaCl and water, large amounts would be lost in the urine. If such an increase in excretion were not accompanied by a corresponding rise in dietary intake, the organism would develop a negative NaCl and water balance. Therefore, glomerulotubular balance helps maintain NaCl and water homeostasis despite changes in GFR and the filtered load of water and NaCl.

8. See Table 4-6.

■ CHAPTER 5

1. This problem illustrates the importance of effective vs. ineffective osmoles in regulating ADH secretion. Although plasma osmolality is elevated, the increased osmolality is due to urea. Because urea is an ineffective osmole with regard to ADH secretion, it is necessary to estimate the osmolality of plasma that is due to effective osmoles (Na^+ and its anions). The effective osmolality of the plasma is estimated by doubling the plasma [Na^+], which yields a value of 270 mOsm/kg H_2O. Because the effective osmolality is reduced from normal (normal = 280 to 290 mOsm/kg H_2O), ADH secretion is suppressed and plasma levels are reduced.

2. see table below

Tubular fluid osmolality is the same, regardless of the presence of ADH, in all segments except the collecting duct. When ADH is present, the tubular fluid within the lumen of the collecting duct comes to osmotic equilibrium with the surrounding interstitial fluid (300 mOsm/kg H_2O in the cortex and 1,200 mOsm/kg H_2O in the medulla). In the absence of ADH, solute reabsorption along the collecting duct leads to further dilution of the tubular fluid.

3. a. The first step in calculating free-water clearance is to calculate the osmolar clearance (C_{osm}):

$$C_{osm} = \frac{U_{osm} \times \dot{V}}{P_{osm}}$$

$$= \frac{70 \text{ mOsm/kg } H_2O \times 3 \text{ ml/min}}{295 \text{ mOsm/kg } H_2O} = 0.7 \text{ ml/min}$$

C_{H_2O} is then calculated as:

$$C_{H_2O} = \dot{V} - C_{osm} = 3 \text{ ml/min} - 0.7 \text{ ml/min} = 2.3 \text{ ml/min}$$

b. In this example:

$$C_{osm} = \frac{U_{osm} \times \dot{V}}{P_{osm}}$$

$$= \frac{1,100 \text{ mOsm/kg } H_2O \times 0.4 \text{ ml/min}}{295 \text{ mOsm/kg } H_2O} = 1.5 \text{ ml/min}$$

C_{H_2O} is then calculated as:

$$C_{H_2O} = \dot{V} - C_{osm} = 0.4 \text{ ml/min} - 1.5 \text{ ml/min}$$
$$= -1.1 \text{ ml/min } (T^c_{H_2O})$$

4. a. *Decreased renal perfusion:* With a decrease in renal perfusion, as would occur

Nephron site	0-ADH	Maximum ADH
Proximal tubule	300	300
Beginning of thin descending limb	300	300
Beginning of thin ascending limb	1,200	1,200
End of thick ascending limb	≈100	≈100
End of cortical collecting duct	<100	300
Urine	≈50	1,200

with contraction of the effective circulating volume, there is reduced delivery of solute and water to Henle's loop (GFR is decreased, therefore filtered load is decreased and proximal tubule functional reabsorption is enhanced). As a result, there is less separation of solute and water, and $T^c_{H_2O}$ is reduced.

b. *Inhibition of thick ascending limb transport:* Inhibition of thick ascending limb NaCl transport decreases the separation of solute and water that occurs at this site. Because transport by the thick ascending limb is necessary for the generation of the medullary interstitial osmotic gradient, the osmolality of the interstitium will fall. This impairs the reabsorption of water from the medullary collecting duct. As a result, $T^c_{H_2O}$ is reduced. The urine osmolality will approach 300 mOsm/kg H_2O, reflecting the fact that fluid entering Henle's loop from the proximal tubule has an osmolality of this value, and separation of solute and water is impaired.

c. *Nephrogenic diabetes insipidus:* In nephrogenic diabetes insipidus, the collecting duct does not respond to ADH. As a result, it remains impermeable to water. This obviously impairs the ability of the kidneys to concentrate the urine and reabsorb solute-free water ($T^c_{H_2O}$).

5. If daily solute excretion is 800 mOsm, and the individual can only produce concentrated urine with an osmolality of 400 mOsm/kg H_2O, the minimum volume of urine required for this solute excretion is:

$$\frac{800 \text{ mOsm}}{400 \text{ mOsm/kg } H_2O} = 2 \text{ L}$$

If insensible loss is 1 L, this individual must drink at least 3 L of water (or another dilute beverage) in that 24-hour period to prevent the development of hyperosmolality. This is slightly more than the average daily intake of most individuals. For the second individual, the daily water requirement is much less, because of the ability to excrete a more concentrated urine. Minimum urine volume required in this individual would be:

$$\frac{800 \text{ mOsm}}{1,200 \text{ mOsm/kg } H_2O} = 0.67 \text{ L}$$

With insensible loss of 1 L, daily water intake could be less than 2 L, and body fluid osmolality would be maintained. A corollary to these examples is that solute excretion also places constraints on the maximum volume of water that can be ingested. For example, if an individual who can dilute urine to 100 mOsm/kg H_2O excretes 800 mOsm of solute, this person could drink as much as 8 L of water without reducing body fluid osmolality. If, however, the individual excretes more solute (e.g., 1,200 mOsm) 12 L of water could be ingested. Indeed, a decline in body fluid osmolality can be seen in individuals who drink large quantities of water without sufficient solute intake.

■ CHAPTER 6

1. It is assumed that the 3 kg weight loss reflects loss of fluid. Since plasma [Na^+] is unchanged, this represents a loss of isotonic fluid (3 L) from the ECF.

Plasma osmolality: Because plasma [Na^+] is unchanged, the plasma osmolality is unchanged.

Effective circulating volume (ECV): The loss of fluid from the ECF will decrease the effective circulating volume.

ADH secretion: The decrease in ECV, through the vascular baroreceptors, will stimulate ADH secretion.

Urine osmolality: The increased levels of ADH will lead to water conservation by the kidneys, and a concentrated urine will be excreted.

Sensation of thirst: Again, the decrease in ECV, through the vascular baroreceptors, will lead to an enhanced sensation of thirst.

2. The individual is euvolemic. To remain in Na$^+$ balance, the amount of Na$^+$ ingested in the diet must equal the amount excreted from the body. Because the kidneys are the primary route for Na$^+$ excretion, the amount of Na$^+$ excreted daily is nearly equal to the amount ingested in the diet (small amounts of Na$^+$ are lost in perspiration and feces). Therefore, the Na$^+$ excretion rate in this individual is approximately 200 mEq/day.

3.

Regulatory factor	Increased ECV	Decreased ECV
Renal sympathetic nerves	↓	↑
ANP	↑	↓
Renin-angiotensin	↓	↑
Aldosterone	↓	↑
Vasopressin	↓	↑

4. This individual has gained 4 kg. This represents the accumulation of 4 L of fluid (1 kg = 1 L) in the ECF, a portion of which will accumulate in the interstitial fluid compartment as edema. The composition of this fluid is the same as plasma and has an [Na$^+$] of 145 mEq/L. Recall that the accumulation of the fluid requires Na$^+$ retention by the kidney. Therefore, the amount of Na$^+$ retained by the kidney must equal the amount contained in 4 L of fluid having a [Na$^+$] of 145 mEq/L, or 580 mEq of Na$^+$.

5. Aldosterone stimulates Na$^+$ reabsorption in the collecting duct, which explains the reduction in Na$^+$ excretion seen during the beginning of aldosterone treatment. As a result of the positive Na$^+$ balance, the effective circulating volume is increased. This in turn reduces proximal tubule reabsorption and enhances delivery of Na$^+$ to the collecting duct. Additionally, ANP levels are increased, and its action on the collecting duct to inhibit Na$^+$ reabsorption, together with increased Na$^+$ delivery, results in the return of Na$^+$ excretion to its previous level. A new steady state is reached in which ECV is expanded and body weight is increased, reflecting the increased volume of the extracellular fluid compartment. With cessation of aldosterone treatment, the Na$^+$ reabsorptive rate of the collecting duct decreases. Because of the increased ECV and therefore enhanced Na$^+$ delivery to the collecting duct, the reabsorptive capacity of the collecting duct is overwhelmed, and Na$^+$ excretion increases. After a period of negative Na$^+$ balance, the ECV decreases back to normal. A new steady state is reached, and body weight returns to its original value as the extracellular fluid volume decreases.

■ CHAPTER 7

1. Intravenous infusion of K$^+$ into a subject with a combination of sympathetic blockade and insulin deficiency would result in significant hyperkalemia compared with a similar infusion of K$^+$ in a normal subject. Although aldosterone secretion would be stimulated by the hyperkalemia, this hormone stimulates cell K$^+$ uptake after a one-hour lag period. In the first hour following K$^+$ infusion, less than 50% of the infused K$^+$ is excreted by the kidneys, and, because sympathetic activity and insulin release are suppressed, most of the K$^+$ left in the body will remain in the extracellular fluid.

2. Aldosterone deficiency would initially reduce urinary potassium excretion, and K$^+$ would be retained in the body (i.e., dietary intake would exceed excretion). This would lead to hyperkalemia, which is a potent stimulus of K$^+$ excretion. Because the individual is initially in positive K$^+$ balance, plasma K$^+$ rises until urinary K$^+$ excretion equals dietary K$^+$ intake. In the new steady state, K$^+$ intake would equal K$^+$ excretion, although the subject has hyperkalemia. Thus, it is possible to match dietary K$^+$ intake with excretion in the absence of aldosterone; however, this occurs at an elevated plasma [K$^+$].

3. In the first hour after a meal, the rise in plasma K^+ is blunted by the rapid (minutes) uptake of K^+ into skeletal muscle, liver, bone, and red blood cells. Some K^+ is excreted by the kidneys, but, in the first hour following the meal, most K^+ is sequestered in the intracellular fluid. In the ensuing hours, K^+ slowly leaves the cells and is excreted by the kidneys, thus maintaining K^+ balance and plasma $[K^+]$.

4. K^+ excretion is determined primarily by the rate of K^+ secretion by the distal tubule and collecting duct, and is largely independent of the filtered load of K^+. Thus, changes in GFR do not have an appreciable effect on urinary K^+ excretion.

■ CHAPTER 8

1. If urinary buffers were not available, the 70 mEq of acid the kidney needs to excrete to maintain acid-base balance (net acid excretion = nonvolatile acid production), would have to be excreted as free H^+. If the minimum urine pH is 4.0, this represents only 0.1 mEq/L of H^+. Thus, to excrete 70 mEq of H^+, the daily urine output would need to be:

$$\frac{70 \text{ mEq/day}}{0.1 \text{ mEq/L}} = 700 \text{ L}$$

This exceeds the daily glomerular filtration rate (180 L/day). Thus, the urinary buffers are essential for the kidney's ability to excrete sufficient quantities of H^+ to maintain acid-base balance.

2. see table below

The first six disorders are simple acid-base disorders. The last two represent mixed disorders. Mixed metabolic and respiratory acidosis is seen during cardiopulmonary arrest. With cessation of cardiac function, the tissues are inadequately perfused and resort to anaerobic metabolism (production of lactic acid). With cessation of respiration, there is also CO_2 retention. In the example of mixed metabolic acidosis and respiratory alkalosis, pH is normal, but both the $[HCO_3^-]$ and P_{CO_2} are abnormal. An example of a clinical condition producing such a disorder is an overdose of aspirin. The metabolic acidosis is the result of the salicylic acid (active ingredient of aspirin), and the respiratory alkalosis is the result of hyperventilation secondary to salicylic acid stimulation of the respiratory centers.

3. The initial set of laboratory data indicates the presence of a metabolic alkalosis with appropriate respiratory compensation. Given the individual's history, the most likely cause of this simple acid-base disorder is the loss of gastric acid by vomiting. The second set of laboratory data continues to show a metabolic alkalosis with respiratory compensation. In addition, there is evidence of fluid loss (decrease in body weight by 2 kg) and, as a result, a contracted ECV (decrease in blood pressure). Given the worsening of this individual's metabolic alkalosis, it is somewhat

pH	$[HCO_3^-]$, mEq/L	P_{CO_2}, mm Hg	Disorder
7.34	15	29	Metabolic acidosis
7.49	35	48	Metabolic alkalosis
7.47	14	20	Chronic respiratory alkalosis
7.34	31	60	Chronic respiratory acidosis
7.26	26	60	Acute respiratory acidosis
7.62	20	20	Acute respiratory alkalosis
7.09	15	50	Metabolic + respiratory acidosis
7.40	15	25	Metabolic acidosis + respiratory alkalosis

surprising that the urine pH is so acidic. The appropriate renal response should be an increase in HCO_3^- excretion to correct the alkalosis. However, by decreasing the filtered load of HCO_3^- (decreased GFR) and stimulating proximal Na^+ reabsorption, the decreased ECV prevents the excretion of HCO_3^- (HCO_3^- reabsorption is linked to Na^+). To correct this situation, the ECV must be restored to its normal value. Infusion of isotonic NaCl would accomplish this and also allow the kidneys to excrete the excess HCO_3^-, thereby restoring acid-base balance.

4. Carbonic anhydrase plays a critical role in the reabsorption of HCO_3^- by the cells of the proximal tubule and the intercalated cells of the collecting duct. Inhibition of this enzyme would therefore inhibit the reabsorption of HCO_3^- at these nephron sites. Due to the large fraction of the filtered load of HCO_3^- reabsorbed by the proximal tubule, the effect at this site is quantitatively more important. With decreased reabsorption, more HCO_3^- would be excreted in the urine, and urine pH would become alkaline. This loss of HCO_3^- from the body would result in the development of a metabolic acidosis.

■ CHAPTER 9

1. Approximately two thirds of Ca^{++} reabsorption across the proximal tubule occurs by solvent drag, a process that depends on Na^+ reabsorption. Mannitol would inhibit Ca^{++} reabsorption by blocking solvent drag in the proximal tubule and thereby increase urinary Ca^{++} excretion.

2. Furosemide would inhibit the $1Na^+, 2Cl^-$, $1K^+$ symporter and reduce the lumen-positive transepithelial voltage to zero. This in turn would inhibit passive Ca^{++} reabsorption via the paracellular pathway.

3. A rise in plasma $[PO_4^{3-}]$ above 2 mEq/L increases the filtered load of PO_4^{3-} to a value that exceeds the T_m for PO_4^{3-} reabsorption by the nephron. Therefore, PO_4^{3-} excretion

increases and exceeds absorption by the gastrointestinal tract. This produces a negative PO_4^{3-} balance and reduces plasma $[PO_4^{3-}]$.

■ CHAPTER 10

1. see table on p. 180
To determine the type of diuretic, its effect on both C_{H_2O} and $T^c_{H_2O}$ must be determined.
Diuretic A: Diuretic A increases both C_{H_2O} and $T^c_{H_2O}$. This diuretic must be acting proximal to the thick ascending limb of Henle's loop. By inhibiting Na^+ transport at a site proximal to the thick ascending limb, the delivery of solute and water to the thick ascending limb is increased. With increased delivery, there is increased separation of solute and water, which increases both C_{H_2O} and $T^c_{H_2O}$. Diuretic A could be either an osmotic diuretic or a carbonic anhydrase inhibitor.
Diuretic B: Diuretic B inhibits both C_{H_2O} and $T^c_{H_2O}$. Therefore, it must be acting on a nephron site that separates solute from water. In addition, at least a portion of this nephron segment must be in the medulla to account for the decrease in $T^c_{H_2O}$. This nephron site is the thick ascending limb of Henle's loop. By separating solute from water at this site, it contributes to the generation of C_{H_2O}. It also contributes to the maintenance of the medullary interstitial osmotic gradient and thus $T^c_{H_2O}$. Diuretic B is a loop diuretic (e.g., furosemide, ethacrynic acid, bumetanide).
Diuretic C: Diuretic C inhibits C_{H_2O}, but has no effect on $T^c_{H_2O}$. This diuretic must be acting in the cortex to inhibit the separation of solute and water. Both thiazide diuretics and K^+-sparing diuretics act in the cortex. However, K^+-sparing diuretics do not have an appreciable effect on C_{H_2O} (the magnitude of Na^+ transport inhibited by K^+-sparing diuretics is too small). Therefore, diuretic C must be a thiazide diuretic (e.g., chlorothiazide, metolazone).

2. Nephrogenic diabetes insipidus is a condition in which the collecting duct does not

Condition	P_{osm} (mOsm/kg H_2O)	U_{osm} (mOsm/kg H_2O)	$\dot{V}$ (ml/min)	C_{H_2O} (ml/min)	$T^c_{H_2O}$ (ml/min)
Water diuresis					
Before diuretic A	285	70	10	7.54	
After diuretic A	284	125	16	8.96	
Before diuretic B	286	65	12	9.27	
After diuretic B	286	200	19	5.71	
Before diuretic C	284	70	11	8.29	
After diuretic C	285	195	15	4.74	
Antidiuresis					
Before diuretic A	288	1,200	0.6		1.90
After diuretic A	289	450	12.0		6.69
Before diuretic B	290	1,100	0.7		1.96
After diuretic B	288	300	13.0		0.54
Before diuretic C	287	1,200	0.7		2.23
After diuretic C	290	355	10.0		2.24

respond to ADH. As a result, water cannot be reabsorbed, and large volumes of dilute urine are excreted. The key to understanding how long-term thiazide diuretic therapy can lead to a reduction in urine excretion with this condition is the fact that this therapy leads to a reduction in ECV. With this decrease in ECV, there is enhanced reabsorption of solute and water by the proximal tubule. As a result, less fluid is delivered to Henle's loop and thereby into the water-impermeable collecting duct. With this decreased distal delivery of fluid, urine volume is reduced, even though the collecting duct cannot reabsorb water. The thiazide diuretic does not correct the underlying cause of nephrogenic diabetes insipidus, but does provide symptomatic relief from the polyuria. The beneficial effect of the thiazide diuretic can be negated if the ECV is allowed to re-expand, e.g., by the ingestion of large quantities of Na^+.

3. a. The long-term effect of diuretic therapy is the reduction of the ECV. With such a decrease, the blood volume and thus cardiac output are reduced. Because blood pressure is equal to cardiac output times the total peripheral vascular resistance, a decrease in cardiac output reduces pressure. Additionally, diuretics may cause some degree of vascular smooth muscle vasodilation, although the mechanism by which this occurs is not fully understood. This vasodilation reduces total peripheral vascular resistance, thereby decreasing blood pressure.

b. Hypokalemia is a side effect of all diuretics acting proximal to the K^+ secretory site (distal tubule and cortical collecting duct). The most common diuretics given for the treatment of hypertension are thiazides. However, loop diuretics, osmotic diuretics, and carbonic anhydrase inhibitors can also lead to hypokalemia. By their action, flow rate and Na^+ delivery to the K^+ secretory site is enhanced, which in turn stimulates K^+ secretion. Additionally, the diuretic-induced decrease in ECV leads to stimulation of aldosterone secretion by the adrenal cortex via the renin-angiotensin system. Aldosterone also directly stimulates K^+ secretion by the distal tubule and cortical collecting duct.

c. Treatment of the hypokalemia could involve supplementing the diet with foods containing high levels of K^+ or with KCl tablets. Alternatively, a K^+-sparing diuretic could be given in combination with the thiazide diuretic.

4. Thiazide diuretics are secreted into the lumen of the proximal tubule by the same organic anion transport system that secretes penicillin. Competitive inhibition of secretion of the thiazide could decrease the effective concentration of the diuretic in the tubular fluid. Since thiazides act from the lumen, a reduction in their concentration at this site could reduce their effectiveness.

Review Examination

1. Through metabolism, an individual produces 900 mOsm/day of solute, which must be excreted by the kidneys. If this individual has a urine concentrating defect and can only produce urine with a maximum osmolality of 300 mOsm/kg H_2O, what is the minimum volume of water that must be ingested to prevent a rise in body fluid osmolality? Assume that insensible water loss is 1.5 L.
   a. 1.5 L.
   b. 3.0 L.
   c. 4.5 L.
   d. 6.0 L.

2. Three individuals, each weighing 55 kg and having a plasma $[Na^+]$ of 145 mEq/L, are infused with different solutions. Individual A is infused with 1 L of isotonic NaCl (290 mOsm/kg H_2O); individual B is infused with 1 L of a mannitol solution (290 mOsm/kg H_2O; and individual C is infused with 1 L of a urea solution (290 mOsm/kg H_2O). Assuming there is no urine output, which of these individuals will have a lower plasma $[Na^+]$ after complete equilibration of the ECF an ICF?
   a. Individual A (NaCl infusion).
   b. Individual B (mannitol infusion).
   c. Individual C (urea infusion).

3. Proximal tubule reabsorption of Na^+ is increased by all of the following *except*:
   a. Contraction of the effective circulating volume.
   b. An increase in the peritubular oncotic pressure.
   c. An increase in renal sympathetic nerve activity.
   d. Elevated levels of aldosterone.

For questions 4 through 6, consider the following graph, which shows the relationship between plasma [PAH] and PAH secretion:

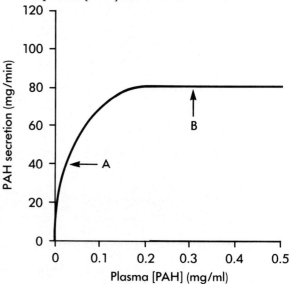

4. The amount of PAH filtered at the glomerulus is:
   a. Greater at point A than at point B.
   b. Less at point A than at point B.
   c. The same at points A and B.

5. The amount of PAH excreted in the urine is:
   a. Greater at point A than at point B.
   b. Less at point A than at point B.
   c. The same at points A and B.

6. The clearance of PAH is:
   a. Greater at point A than at point B.
   b. Less at point A than at point B.
   c. The same at points A and B.

7. You wish to determine how substance x is handled by the kidneys. You know that 25% of substance x is bound to plasma protein. The following data are obtained:

   Clearance of inulin = 120 ml/min
   Plasma [x]　　　　= 0.01 mg/ml
   Urine [x]　　　　 = 1.5 mg/ml
   Urine flow rate　 = 0.6 ml/min

   Substance x is handled by the kidney by:
   a. Filtration alone.
   b. Filtration and reabsorption.
   c. Filtration and secretion.

For questions 8 through 11, match the appropriate diuretic with the statement.
   a. Carbonic anhydrase inhibitor.
   b. Loop diuretic.
   c. Thiazide diuretic.
   d. K^+-sparing diuretic.

8. Administration leads to an increase in the kidneys' ability to excrete solute-free water (C_{H_2O}).

9. Administration may lead to the development of hyperkalemia.

10. Administration impairs the ability of the kidneys to reabsorb solute-free water ($T^c_{H_2O}$).

11. Administration results in a decrease in renal Ca^{++} excretion.

12. An individual suffers from an illness characterized by nausea, vomiting, and diarrhea. Over a two-day period, this individual experiences a 3-kg weight loss without a change in plasma [Na^+]. Which of the following statements is *true?*
    a. The volume of ICF is unchanged.
    b. The volume of ECF is decreased.
    c. Total body osmoles are reduced.
    d. Plasma osmolality is unchanged.
    e. All of the above are true.

13. Hyponatremia (i.e., reduced plasma [Na^+]) can be seen in individuals whose effective circulating volume is decreased. Which of the following factors contributes to the development of hyponatremia in this situation?
    a. Impaired ability of the kidneys to excrete solute-free water (C_{H_2O}).
    b. Elevated levels of atrial natriuretic peptide (ANP).
    c. Increased excretion of Na^+ by the kidneys.
    d. Decreased levels of antidiuretic hormone (ADH).

14. An individual weighs 60 kg and ingests a diet containing 100 mEq/day of Na^+. This individual is placed on a thiazide diuretic. After two months on this diuretic and with no change in diet, which of the following statements is *true?*
    a. Body weight is less than 60 kg.
    b. Urine Na^+ excretion is greater than 100 mEq/day.
    c. Plasma aldosterone levels are suppressed.
    d. Plasma [Na^+] is reduced.

15. All of the following statements concerning the defense of body fluid pH after an acute infusion of acid are true *except:*
    a. Some of the acid is buffered by the extracellular HCO_3^-.
    b. The ventilatory rate is rapidly (minutes to hours) increased.
    c. Some of the acid is buffered intracellularly.

    d. There is a rapid (minutes to hours) increase in renal ammoniagenesis and acid excretion.

16. Production of a concentrated urine (U_{osm} = 1,200 mOsm/kg H_2O) requires which of the following?

    a. Presence of ADH.

    b. Active NaCl reabsorption by the thick ascending limb of Henle's loop.

    c. Medullary hyperosmolality of at least 1,200 mOsm/kg H_2O.

    d. Collecting duct responsive to ADH.

    e. All of the above.

17. Inhibition of carbonic anhydrase would be expected to result in all of the following *except:*

    a. Development of a metabolic acidosis.

    b. Inhibition of HCO_3^- reabsorption by the proximal tubule.

    c. Increase in pH of fluid within the lumen of the collecting duct.

    d. Increase in the filtered load of HCO_3^-.

18. A decrease in effective circulating volume will result in the enhanced proximal tubule reabsorption of which of the following substances?

    a. Na^+.

    b. HCO_3^-.

    c. PO_4^{3-}.

    d. Ca^{++}.

    e. All of the above.

19. The volume of plasma from which all of a substance is removed (per unit time) and excreted into the urine is termed:

    a. The renal plasma flow.

    b. The glomerular filtration rate.

    c. The renal clearance.

    d. The filtration fraction.

    e. None of the above.

Assign the appropriate diagnosis from those listed below to the conditions described in questions 20 through 24.

    a. Metabolic acidosis with respiratory compensation.

    b. Metabolic alkalosis with respiratory compensation.

    c. Respiratory acidosis with renal compensation (chronic respiratory acidosis).

    d. Respiratory acidosis without renal compensation (acute respiratory acidosis).

    e. Metabolic acidosis and respiratory acidosis.

Use the following normal values:

pH   = 7.40

$[HCO_3^-]$ = 24 mEq/L

Pco_2 = 40 mm Hg

20. An individual with an asthma attack:

    pH = 7.32; $[HCO_3^-]$ = 25 mEq/L; Pco_2 = 50 mm Hg.

21. An individual with diabetes mellitus who forgets to take insulin:

    pH = 7.29; $[HCO_3^-]$ = 12 mEq/L; Pco_2 = 26 mm Hg.

22. An individual in cardiopulmonary arrest:

    pH = 6.85; $[HCO_3^-]$ = 10 mEq/L; Pco_2 = 60 mm Hg.

23. An individual with a gastric ulcer who ingests large quantities of antacids:

    pH = 7.45; $[HCO_3^-]$ = 30 mEq/L; Pco_2 = 45 mm Hg.

24. An individual with a 20-year history of smoking three packs/day who has emphysema:

    pH = 7.37; $[HCO_3^-]$ = 28 mEq/L; Pco_2 = 50 mm Hg.

25. An individual is found to have a T_m for glucose of 400 mg/min and an inulin clearance of 100 ml/min. What is the plasma threshold for glucose in this individual?

    a. 0.04 mg/ml.

    b. 0.4 mg/ml.

    c. 4 mg/ml.

    d. 40 mg/ml.

26. Proximal tubule HCO_3^- reabsorption is inhibited by:

    a. Increased Pco_2.

    b. Expansion of the ECV.

    c. Systemic acidosis.

d. Decreased levels of aldosterone.

e. None of the above.

27. Renal NH_4^+ excretion is increased under which of the following conditions?

a. Systemic acidosis.

b. Low urine pH.

c. Ingestion of a diet producing large amounts of nonvolatile acid.

d. Hypokalemia.

e. All of the above.

28. An individual is infused with 80 mg of inulin to determine the volume of the ECF compartment. After equilibration, a blood sample is obtained, and the plasma [inulin] is 5 mg/L. What is the volume of the ECF compartment (assume no inulin excretion)?

a. 8 L.

b. 12 L.

c. 14 L.

d. 16 L.

29. Substance Y is handled by the kidneys by filtration and reabsorption. As plasma [Y] is increased, all of the following occur *except:*

a. The T_m for Y decreases.

b. The excretion rate of Y increases.

c. The filtered load of Y increases.

d. The clearance of Y increases.

30. Aldosterone has which of the following actions?

a. Stimulates Na^+ reabsorption by the principal cell of the collecting duct.

b. Stimulates the uptake of K^+ into cells (e.g., skeletal muscle).

c. Stimulates H^+ secretion by intercalated cells of the collecting duct.

d. Stimulates K^+ secretion by the principal cell of the collecting duct.

e. All of the above.

31. ADH secretion is stimulated by all of the following *except:*

a. Infusion of hypertonic NaCl.

b. Infusion of a urea solution.

c. Contraction of the ECV.

d. Deprivation of water intake for 24 hours.

32. Which of the following statements about renal Na^+ excretion is *false?*

a. In the steady state, renal Na^+ excretion equals Na^+ ingestion.

b. The collecting duct makes small adjustments in renal Na^+ excretion during euvolemia.

c. The delivery of Na^+ to the collecting duct is constant under all conditions.

d. Aldosterone decreases renal Na^+ excretion.

33. Metabolism of all of the following food stuffs will produce nonvolatile acid *except:*

a. Sulfur-containing amino acids.

b. Cationic amino acids.

c. Organic anions.

d. Anaerobic metabolism of glucose.

e. Fat metabolism in the absence of insulin.

34. Which of the following statements about renin release from the juxtaglomerular apparatus is *false?*

a. Increased delivery of NaCl to the macula densa increases renin secretion.

b. A reduction in renal perfusion pressure increases renin secretion.

c. Inhibition of converting enzyme (i.e., block conversion of angiotensin I to angiotensin II) increases renin secretion.

d. Stimulation of renal sympathetic nerve fibers increases renin secretion.

35. Renal PO_4^{3-} excretion is enhanced by which of the following?

a. PTH.

b. Expansion of the ECF.

c. Infusion of an osmotic diuretic.

d. All of the above.

36. Which of the following statements about renal Ca^{++} handling is *false?*

a. The largest fraction of the filtered load of Ca^{++} is reabsorbed in the proximal tubule.

b. PTH stimulates Ca^{++} reabsorption in the distal tubule.

c. Proximal tubule Ca^{++} reabsorption is enhanced when the ECF is contracted.

d. Thiazide diuretics increase Ca^{++} excretion.

e. Loop diuretics increase Ca^{++} excretion.

37. Which of the following structures are part of the glomerular filtration barrier?
    a. Fenestrated endothelium.
    b. Glomerular basement membrane.
    c. Visceral epithelial cells (podocytes).
    d. All of the above.

38. All of the following *except* one is a component of the juxtaglomerular apparatus:
    a. Macula densa.
    b. Extraglomerular mesangial cells.
    c. Renin-producing granular cells.
    d. Angiotensin-producing cells.

39. The driving force for passive reabsorption of Na^+ in the *late* proximal tubule is:
    a. Higher luminal than peritubular hydrostatic pressure.
    b. Higher luminal than peritubular $[Na^+]$.
    c. Lumen-positive potential established by passive reabsorption of Cl^-.
    d. Lumen-positive potential established by active reabsorption of HCO_3^-.

40. Na^+ reabsorption by the thick ascending limb of Henle's loop is:
    a. Regulated by Starling forces.
    b. Inhibited by angiotensin II.
    c. Increased with increased delivered load of Na^+.
    d. Inhibited by K^+-sparing diuretics.

41. Which nephron segment contributes most to potassium excretion when dietary potassium is altered?
    a. Proximal convoluted tubule.
    b. Descending limb of Henle's loop.
    c. Proximal straight tubule.
    d. Distal tubule.
    e. Thick ascending limb of Henle's loop.

42. According to the tubuloglomerular feedback theory, an increase in the flow of tubular fluid to the macula densa will result in:

a. A decrease in the glomerular filtration rate of the same nephron.

b. An increase in renal blood flow.

c. Activation of the renal sympathetic nerves.

d. An increase in proximal tubule solute and water reabsorption.

43. A drug increases the glomerular filtration rate. The drug may act by:
    a. Increasing the ultrafiltration coefficient, K_f.
    b. Constricting the afferent arterioles.
    c. Decreasing renal blood flow.
    d. Increasing plasma protein concentration.

44. During antidiuresis, tubular fluid is hyperosmotic to plasma in the following parts of the nephron:
    a. Thick ascending limb of Henle's loop.
    b. Distal tubule.
    c. Bend of Henle's loop.
    d. Bowman's space.

45. Potassium excretion is enhanced by:
    a. Mannitol diuresis.
    b. Acute metabolic acidosis.
    c. Hypoaldosteronism.
    d. Decreased tubular flow rate.

46. Water reabsorption by the proximal tubule is:
    a. Against its concentration gradient.
    b. Dependent upon Na^+ reabsorption.
    c. Regulated by aldosterone.
    d. Not affected by Starling forces.

47. During a 24-hour period, an individual excretes in the urine 60 mmol of NH_4^+, 40 mmol of T.A., and 10 mmol of HCO_3^-. If this individual is in acid-base balance, how much nonvolatile acid was produced from metabolism?
    a. 90 mmol/day.
    b. 100 mmol/day.
    c. 110 mmol/day.
    d. None of the above.

48. Infusion of 1 L of which of the following

solutions will lead to the largest increase in ECF volume?

a. Water.
b. Isotonic NaCl.
c. Hypotonic NaCl.
d. Hypertonic NaCl.

49. The rate of ultrafiltration across glomerular capillaries is higher than ultrafiltration across other capillaries in the body because:

a. The hydrostatic pressure is higher in glomerular capillaries than in other capillaries.
b. The oncotic pressure is higher in glomerular capillaries than in other capillaries.
c. The ultrafiltration coefficient is 100 times higher in glomerular capillaries than in other capillaries.
d. The oncotic pressure in Bowman's space is lower than that in the interstitium surrounding other capillaries.

50. All of the following are actions of angiotensin II *except*:

a. Stimulates thirst.
b. Inhibits renin secretion.
c. Stimulates aldosterone secretion from the adrenal cortex.
d. Inhibits proximal tubule Na^+ reabsorption.

■ ANSWERS

1. c	26. b
2. b	27. e
3. d	28. d
4. b	29. a
5. b	30. e
6. a	31. b
7. a	32. c
8. a	33. c
9. d	34. a
10. b	35. d
11. c	36. d
12. e	37. d
13. a	38. d
14. a	39. c
15. d	40. c
16. e	41. d
17. d	42. a
18. e	43. a
19. c	44. c
20. d	45. a
21. a	46. b
22. e	47. a
23. b	48. d
24. c	49. c
25. c	50. d

Index

A

Acid, metabolic production of, 124-125*t*

Acid-base balance, 123
analysis of acid-base disorders, 137-138, 137*f*
CO_2/HCO_3^- buffer system, 123-124
effect of, on K^+ secretion, 121-122
formation of new HCO_3^-, 129-130*f*, 131*f*, 132
HCO_3^- reabsorption along the nephron, 127-128*f*, 127*f*
regulation of, 128-129, 134*t*
and internal K^+ distribution, 114
renal acid excretion, 125-126

Acid-base disorders
analysis of, 137-138, 137*f*
characteristics of, 135*t*
metabolic acidosis, 135-136
metabolic alkalosis, 136
respiratory acidosis, 136
respiratory alkalosis, 136-137
response to, 132-133
extracellular and intracellular buffering, 133-134
renal defense, 134-135*t*
respiratory defense, 134

Acidosis, 132

Active transport mechanisms, 50

Adenylyl cyclase, 76

Addison's disease, 114, 150

Adrenergic fibers, 24

α-adrenergic receptors, 25

Afferent arteriole, 16

Albumin, reabsorption by proximal tubule, 38

Aldosterone
actions of, 157, 177, 181
deficiency of, 177
effect of, on K^+ secretion, 119*f*
and internal K^+ distribution, 114
as regulatory factor for HCO_3^- reabsorption, 129
secretion of, 23
and stimulation of Na^+ reabsorption, 95-96

Aldosterone-induced proteins, 96

Aldosteronism, 114

Alkali, metabolic production of, 124-125*t*

Alkalosis, 132

ρ-Aminohippuric acid (PAH)
clearance of, 32-33, 34*f*, 35*f*
relationship between renal plasma flow and, 36

Ammonia (NH_3/NH_4^+), 126
in formation of new HCO_3^-, 129-130, 132

Angiotensin I, 95

Angiotensin II, 23, 95
and regulation of renal blood flow, 46-47, 46*f*

Angiotensinogen, 94-95

Antidiuresis, 71

Antidiuretic hormone (ADH), 71-72*f*, 97
actions on kidney, 75-76
disorders of secretion and action, 76
effect of, on K^+ secretion, 120*f*, 121
hemodynamic control of secretion, 73*f*, 74-75, 74*f*
osmotic control of secretion, 72, 73*f*, 74

Antidiuretic hormone—cont'd
role of, and diuresis versus antidiuresis, 80*f*, 83
secretion of, 176
by the posterior pituitary, 72

Antiport, 51

Arcuate artery, 16

Arcuate vein, 16

Atrial natriuretic peptide, 93, 97

Autoregulation, of glomerular filtration rate, 45, 99-100

B

Baroreceptors, 74-75, 93

Basement membrane, 19, 22

Basolateral membrane, 18

Bladder, 16, 24
innervation of, 25
passage of urine from pelvis to, 25
volume of, 24-25

Body fluid(s)
capillary fluid exchange, 9-10
cellular fluid exchange, 10, 11*f*, 12-13
composition of body fluid compartments, 7-9
fluid exchange between body fluid compartments, 9
measurement of body fluid volumes, 6-7*f*, 6*t*
physicochemical properties of electrolyte solution
molarity and equivalence, 1-2
oncotic pressure, 5*f*
osmolarity and osmolality, 3, 4*t*
osmosis and osmotic pressure, 2-3, 2*t*

Body fluid(s)—cont'd
  physicochemical properties of
      electrolyte solution–cont'd
    specific gravity, 5-6
    tonicity, 3-4
  volumes of body fluid compart-
      ments, 6
Body fluid compartments
  composition of, 7-9
  fluid exchange between, 9
    capillary fluid exchange, 9-10
    cellular fluid exchange, 10,
      11f, 12-13
  volumes of, 6
Body fluid osmolality, 70-71
  antidiuretic hormone,
      71-72f, 71f
    actions on kidneys, 75-76
    disorders of secretion and
        action, 76
    hemodynamic control of
        secretion, 73f, 74-75, 74f
    osmotic control of secretion,
        72, 73f, 74
  countercurrent multiplication
      by Henle's loop,
      77-79, 78f
    diuresis versus antidiuresis,
        80f, 83
    medullary interstitial osmotic
        gradient, 79, 81-82
    transport and permeability
        properties of nephron seg-
        ments, 79, 80f
    vasa recta function, 82-83
  integrated view of the urine
      concentrating process, 83-
      85, 84f
  quantitating renal diluting and
      concentrating ability, 85-
      88, 86f
  thirst, 76-77
Bowman's capsule, 18
  parietal layer of, 19
Bowman's space, 19
  oncotic pressure in, 40, 41f
Brush border, 18

C

Calcium balance (Ca^{++}), 140-141
  body content and distribution
      of, 141t
  excretion of, 161
  forms of, in plasma, 145t

Calcium balance—cont'd
  handling, 160-162
  homeostasis, 141-142, 141f
  reabsorption of, 161
    cellular mechanisms of,
        143-144, 143f
    regulating balance, 140-144
    transport along the nephron,
        142-143
Capillary endothelium, 8
Capillary filtration coefficient, 9
Capillary fluid exchange, 9-10
Capillary hydrostatic pressure,
    106
Capillary permeability, 106
Carbonic anhydrase, 124, 179
Carbonic anhydrase inhibitors,
    156
Celiac plexus, 24
Cell lysis, and internal K^+ distri-
    bution, 115
Cellular fluid exchange, 10, 11f,
    12-13
Central diabetes insipidus, 76
Chemoreceptors, 134
Chlorothiazide, 157
Clearance, 27-29, 28f
  of p-Aminohippuric acid, 32-33,
      34f, 35f
  in estimating transport mecha-
      nism, 36f, 37
  filtration plus tubular secretion,
      32-33, 34f, 35f
  free-water, 85
  of glucose, 31-33
  of inulin, 29-31, 30f
Collecting duct, 170
Compensatory response, analysis
    of, 138
Concentrated urine, 87-88
Converting enzyme, 95
Coronary ischemia, 114
Cortex, 15
Cotransport, 51
Countercurrent exchange, 82-83
Countercurrent flow, 77
Countercurrent multiplier,
    77, 78f
  by Henle's loop, 77-79, 78f,
      80f, 81-83, 82f
Counter-transport, 51
Coupled transport, 51
Creatinine, 30
Cyclic adenosine monophosphate
    (cAMP), 76

D

Detrusor muscle, 24
Dextrans, 38
Diabetes insipidus, 76
  central, 76
  nephrogenic, 76
Diffusion
  facilitated, 51
  passive, 50
Diffusion trapping, 132
1,25-dihydroxyvitamin
    $D_3(1,25(OH)_2D_3)$, 142, 147
Dilute urine, 87
Diluting segment, 79
Distal tubule, 170
  and collecting duct, 62, 64-65
Diuresis, 71
  versus antidiuresis, 80f, 83
Diuretics, 152
  effect of, on the excretion of
      water and other solutes,
      158, 159t
    Ca^{++}, Mg^{++}, and PO_4^{3-} han-
        dling, 160-162
    HCO_3^- handling, 160
    K^+ handling, 159-160
    solute-free water, 158-159
  mechanisms of
    carbonic anhydrase inhibi-
        tors, 156
    K^+-sparing diuretics, 157,
        158f
    loop diuretics, 156-157
    osmotic diuretics, 155-156
    thiazide diuretics, 157
  principles of, 152-155
    adequate delivery of diuretics
        to site of action, 154
    response of more distal
        nephron segments, 153-
        154
    sites of action, 153f
    volume of the ECF, 154-155
Diuretic therapy, long-term effect
    of, 180

E

Edema, 105-106
  role of kidney in, 107-108, 107f
Effective circulating volume
    (ECV), 92, 176
  control of Na^+ excretion
      with decreased, 103-105,
      104f

Effective circulating vol.—cont'd
  control of Na^+ excretion–cont'd
    with increased, 100-103,
      101*f*, 102*f*
    with normal, 97, 98*f*, 99-100
  volume sensors, 92, 93
Effective osmoles, 4, 72
Effective osmotic pressure, 4
Effective renal plasma flow
    (ERPF), 36
Efferent arteriole, 16
Electrolytes, filtration, excretion
    and reabsorption of, 50*t*
Electrolyte solutions
  physicochemical properties of
    molarity and equivalence, 1-2
    oncotic pressure, 5*f*
    osmolarity and osmolality,
      3, 4*t*
    osmosis and osmotic pres-
      sure, 2-3, 2*t*
    specific gravity, 5-6
    tonicity, 3-4
Endocytosis, 52
Epinephrine, and internal K^+ dis-
    tribution, 114
Equivalence, 1-2
Euvolemia, 97
Excretion
  of Ca^{++}, 144
  of Mg^{++}, 146-147
  of PO_4^{3-}, 150
Exercise, and internal K^+ distribu-
    tion, 115
External K^+ balance, 110
External meatus, 24
External sphincter, 24
Extracellular buffering, 133-134
Extracellular fluid, 7
  analysis of fluid shifts
    between, 12
  major solutes in, 90-91
  Na^+ as determinant of osmolal-
    ity, 91
Extracellular fluid volume, 90-91
  control of Na^+ excretion with
    decreased ECV, 103-105,
      104*f*
    with increased ECV, 100-103,
      101*f*, 102*f*
    with normal ECV, 97, 98*f*,
      99-100
  edema and the role of the kid-
    ney, 105-108
  effective circulating volume, 92

Extracellular fluid volume—cont'd
  volume receptor signals, 93
    antidiuretic hormone, 97
    atrial natriuretic peptide, 97
    renal sympathetic nerves,
      93-94
    renin-angiotensin-aldosterone
      system, 94-97, 95*f*, 96*f*
  volume sensors, 92, 93
    vascular high-pressure vol-
      ume receptors, 93
    vascular low-pressure volume
      receptors, 93
Extraglomerular mesangial cells,
    22-23

F

Facilitated diffusion, 51
Filtered load, 31
Filtration barrier, 19, 21*f*, 22
  importance of the negative
    charges on, 40
Filtration fraction, 31
Filtration slits, 22
Free-water clearance, 85
Fundus, 24
Furosemide, 179

G

Glomerular capillaries, 16, 18,
    171
  hydrostatic pressure in, 40, 41*f*
Glomerular filtration
  relationship between molecular
    radius and, 38*t*
  and renal blood flow, 27-47
Glomerular filtration barrier, 38
Glomerular filtration rate
  altering, 42
  autoregulation of, 45, 99-100
  measurement of, 29-31, 30*f*
Glomerulotubular balance, 66-68,
    100, 174-175
  role of, in regulation of NaCl
    and water reabsorption,
    66-68
Glomerulus, 170
  ultrastructure of, 19, 20*f*, 21*f*,
    22-23*f*
Glucose
  clearance of, 31-32
  reabsorption from tubular
    fluid, 31
Glutamine, metabolism by kid-
    neys, 130

Goormaghtigh's cells, 22-23
Granular cells, 23

H

HCO_3^-, 160
  formation of new, 129-130*f*,
    131*f*, 132
  reabsorption along the neph-
    ron, 127-128*f*, 127*f*
Hematocrit (HCT), 36
Hemodynamic control, of ADH
    secretion, 73*f*, 74-75, 74*f*
Henderson-Hasselbalch equation,
    124
Henle's loop, 18, 59-60, 61*f*, 62,
    170
  countercurrent multiplication
    by, 77-79, 78*f*
  diuresis versus antidiuresis
    and the role of ADH,
    80*f*, 83
  medullary interstitial osmotic
    gradient, 79, 81-82
  transport and permeability
    properties of nephron seg-
    ments, 79, 80*f*
  vasa recta function, 82-83
Homeostasis
  Ca^{++}, 141-142, 141*f*
  Mg^{++}, 145-146, 145*f*
  PO_4^{3-}, 147, 148*f*, 149
Hormones, in regulating NaCl and
    water reabsorption, 68*t*
Hypercalcemia, 141
Hyperkalemia, 114, 177
  and aldosterone level, 114
  and cell lysis, 115
  and K^+ balance, 111*f*
  and K^+ secretion, 118
Hyperkalemic individuals, 111
Hypertonic solution, 3
Hypocalcemia, 142
Hypocalcemic tetany, 141
Hypokalemia, 180-181
  and aldosterone level, 114
  effect of, on K^+ secretion, 119
  and K^+ balance, 111*f*
  treatment of, 181
Hypokalemic individual, 111
Hypotonic solution, 3

I

Ineffective osmole, 4, 73, 74
Insensible water loss, 70*n*

Insulin, and internal K^+ distribution, 114
Intercalated cells, 62-63
Interlobar artery, 16
Interlobar vein, 16
Interlobular artery, 16
Interlobular vein, 16
Internal K^+ balance, 110
Internal sphincter, 24
Interstitial fluid, 7
Intracellular buffering, 133-134
Intracellular fluid, 7
  analysis of fluid shifts between, 12
  anion composition of, 9
  composition of, 8-9
Inulin, 29
  clearance of, 29-31, 30f
Isosmotic urine, 86-87
Isotonic solution, 3

J

Juxtaglomerular apparatus, 45, 93, 171
  ultrastructure of, 20f, 23

K

Kidney
  ADH actions on the, 75-76
  in edema formation, 107-108, 107f
  excretion of K^+ by, 115-117, 116f
  excretion of NaCl by, 91-92
  gross anatomy, 15-16f
    glomerulus, 19, 20f, 21f, 22-23f
    juxtaglomerular apparatus, 20f, 23
    nephron, 16, 17f, 18-19f
  innervation of, 24
  and metabolism of glutamine, 130
  in renal water excretion, 70-71

L

Lacis cells, 22-23
Lamina densa and lamina rara externa, 22
Lamina rara interna, 22
Loop diuretics, 156-157, 161
Lymphatic obstruction, 106

M

Macula densa, 18, 23
  delivery of NaCl to the, 94
Magnesium (Mg^{++}), 144
  body content and distribution of, 141t
  excretion, 161
  forms of, in plasma, 145t
  handling, 160-162
  homeostasis, 145-146, 145f
  regulation balance of, 144-147
  regulation of excretion, 146-147
  transport along the nephron, 146f
Major calices, 15
Mass balance, 28
Medulla, 15
Medullary interstitial osmotic gradient, 79, 81-82
Membrane transport, general principles of, 50-52
Mesangial cells, 22
Mesangial matrix, 22
Mesangium, 22
Metabolic acid-base disorders, 124
Metabolic acidosis, 135-136
  effect of on K^+ excretion, 122
  and K^+ level, 114
Metabolic alkalosis, 136
  and K^+ level, 114
Metabolic production of acid and alkali, 124-125t
Metolazone, 157n
Micturition, 25-26, 171
Minor calices, 15
Mixed disorder, 138
Molarity, 1-2
Molecular radius, relationship between glomerular filterability, 38t
Myogenic mechanism, 45

N

Natriuresis, 152, 154
Nephrogenic diabetes insipidus, 76, 176, 179-180
Nephron, 15, 18
  Ca^{++} transport along, 142-143
  Mg^{++} transport along, 146f
  NaCl and water reabsorption along the, 52
    distal tubule and collecting duct, 62, 64-65

Nephron—cont'd
  NaCl and water reabsorption along the—cont'd
    Henle's loop, 59-60, 61f, 62
    proximal tubule, 52, 54-59, 54f, 55f, 56f, 57f, 58t
  $PO_4^{\equiv}$ transport along, 149, 150f
  segments of, 170
    transport and permeability properties of, 79, 80f
  ultrastructure of, 16, 17f, 18-19f
Net acid excretion, 126
Neurohypophysis, 72
Nonionic diffusion, 132
Nonvolatile acids, 125

O

Oncotic pressure, 5f
  peritubular, 65-66
  of plasma proteins, 9
Organic anion
  secretory system, 154
Organic anion secretion, 57
Organic cation secretion, 57-58t
Organic cation secretory systems, 154
Osmolality, 3
  of the tubular fluid, 45
Osmolar clearance, 86
Osmolarity, 3
Osmole
  effective, 4, 72
  ineffective, 4, 73, 74
Osmoreceptors, 72, 73, 74
Osmosis, 2-3, 2t, 50
Osmotic control, of ADH secretion, 72, 73f, 74
Osmotic diuretics, 155-156
Osmotic equilibrium, 10
Osmotic pressure, 3
  differences between extracellular fluid and intracellular fluid, 10
  effective, 4

P

Paracellular pathway, 52, 53f
Parasympathetic fibers, 25
Parathyroid hormone (PTH), 142, 144, 147, 150
Paraventricular nuclei, 72, 75
Passive diffusion, 50

Pelvic space, 15
Pelvis, 15
    passage of urine from, to bladder, 25
Perfusion pressure, 94
Peritubular capillaries, 16
Peritubular oncotic pressure, 65-66
Phosphate PO$_4^{3-}$, 147
    body content and distribution of, 141t
    excretion, 161-162
        regulation of, 150
    forms of, in plasma, 145t
    handling, 160-162
    homeostasis, 147, 148f, 149
    regulating balance, 147-150
    titration curve for, 148
    transport along the nephron, 149, 150f
Plasma, 7
    as determinant of K$^+$ secretion, 118
Plasma oncotic pressure, 106
Plasma osmolality, 175, 176
    estimating, 168
    and internal K$^+$ distribution, 115
Plasma threshold, 31
Podocytes, 19, 22
Pokalemic, 111
Polydipsia, 76
Polyuria, 76
Posterior pituitary, and secretion of ADH, 72
Potassium (K$^+$), 110-112, 111f
    cellular mechanisms of transport by the distal tubule and collecting duct, 117-118, 117f
    diuretics, 157, 158f
    excretion of, by kidneys, 115-117, 116f
    external balance, 115
    internal distribution, 112-113
        acid-base balance, 114
        aldosterone, 114
        cell lysis, 115
        epinephrine, 114
        exercise, 115
        insulin, 114
        plasma osmolality, 115
    regulation of excretion, 118
        acid-base balance, 121-122
        aldosterone, 119f

Potassium (K$^+$)—cont'd
    regulation of excretion—cont'd
        antidiuretic hormone, 120f, 121
        flow rate of tubular fluid, 119
        Na$^+$ of tubular fluid, 122
        plasma, 118-119, 118f
Primary active transport, 174
Principal cells, 62, 63f
Prostaglandins, and regulation of renal blood flow, 47
Protein kinases, 76
Protein reabsorption, 58-59
Proteinuria, 40
Proximal reabsorption, 174
Proximal tubule, 18, 170
    and NaCl and water reabsorption along the nephron, 52, 54-59, 54f, 55f, 56f, 57f, 58t
Proximal tubule HCO$_3^-$ reabsorption, 129
Pudendal nerves, 25

R

Reabsorption
    cellular mechanisms of calcium, 143-144, 143f
    of filtered HCO$_3^-$, 127
Renal acid excretion, 125-126
Renal artery, 16, 28
Renal blood flow, 36, 43f, 44f, 45
    autoregulation of, 45
    glomerular filtration, 27-47
    hormones regulating, 46t
    measurement of, 33-34, 35f, 36-37
    regulation of, 45, 46t
        sympathetic control, 45-46
Renal glomerulus, 18
Renal plasma flow
    measurement of, 33-34, 35f, 36-37
    relationship between PAH clearance, 36
Renal pyramids, 15
Renal sympathetic nerves, 93-94
Renal transport mechanisms
    NaCl and water reabsorption along the nephron, 49-68
        angiotensin II, 46-47, 46f
        prostaglandins, 47
Renal vein, 16
Renin, 23

Renin-angiotensin-aldosterone system, 94-97, 95f, 96f
Respiratory acid-base disorders, 124
Respiratory acidosis, 136
Respiratory alkalosis, 136-137
Respiratory compensation, 135
Rhabdomyolysis, and K$^+$ secretion, 118
Rugae, 24

S

Secondary active transport, 51, 174
Set point, 74, 75
Single effect, 77
Sodium (Na$^+$)
    and determination of ECF osmolality, 91
    delivery
        mechanisms for keeping, to collecting duct constant, 99-100
    excretion
        control of, with decreased ECV, 103-105, 104f
        control of, with increased ECV, 100-103, 101f, 102f
        control of, with normal ECV, 97, 98f, 99-100
    reabsorption
        regulation of collecting duct, 100
        role of aldosterone in, 95-96
Sodium chloride (NaCl), 174
    balance
        negative, 99
        positive, 99
    delivery of, to macula densa, 94
Sodium chloride and water reabsorption, 54-57, 55f
    among nephron
        distal tubule and collecting duct, 62, 64-65
        Henle's loop, 59-60, 61f, 62
        proximal tubule, 52, 54-59, 54f, 55f, 56f, 57f, 58t
    role of ADH in reabsorption, 75
    role of kidneys in excretion of, 90-91
    regulation of
        glomerulotubular balance, 66-68
        hormones, 68t
        Starling forces, 65-66, 67f

Sodium chloride and water reabsorption—cont'd
 regulation of—cont'd
 sympathetic nervous
 system, 68
Solute-free water, excretion from
 body, 85
Solute reabsorption, 59-60, 61*f*
Solutes
 active transport of, 51-52
 filtration, excretion, and reabsorption of, 50*t*
Solvent drag, 51
Specific gravity, 5-6
Splay, 32
Starling forces, 9, 10*f*, 172
 alterations in, 106
 and edema, 105-106
 in regulation of NaCl and water
 reabsorption, 65-66, 67*f*
 and ultrafiltration, 37-38, 41-42
Steady state balance, 155
Supraoptic nuclei, 72, 75
Sympathetic control, in regulation
 of renal blood flow, 45-46
Sympathetic nervous system, in
 regulation of NaCl and water reabsorption, 68
Symport, 51
Syndrome of inappropriate secretion of ADH (SIADH), 76

T

Thiazide diuretics, 157, 161, 181
Thirst, 76-77
 sensation of, 176

Titratable acid, 126
Tonicity, 3-4
Total body water (TBW), 6-7
 calculation of, 168
Total urine output, 87
Transcellular pathway, 52
Transepithelial solute and water
 transport, 52, 53*f*
Trigone, 24
Tritiated water, calculation of,
 168
Tubular fluid
 flow rate of, 119, 120*f*, 121
 Na$^+$ of, 122
Tubular fluid osmolality, 175
Tubular transport maximum, 31
Tubuloglomerular feedback,
 44*f*, 45

U

Ultrafiltrate composition, determinants of, 38, 39*f*, 40
Ultrafiltration, 19
 dynamics of, 40-42, 41*f*
 effect of Starling forces on,
 37-38
Ultrafiltration coefficient, 41
Uniport, 51
Ureters, 15, 24
Urethra, 24
Urinary tract, lower
 gross anatomy and histology,
 24
 innervation of bladder, 25
 micturition, 25-26
 passage of urine from pelvis to
 bladder, 25

Urine
 composition of, 49, 50*t*
 concentrated, 87-88
 dilute, 87
 excretion of hyperosmotic, 77
 formation of, 49
 isosmotic, 86-87
 passage of, from pelvis to bladder, 25
 specific gravity, 6
Urine concentrating process, integrated view of, 83-85, 84*f*
Urine osmolality, 176
Urogenital diaphragm, 24

V

Van't Hoff's law, 3, 5
Vasa recta, 18-19
 function, 82-83
Vasopressin; *see* Antidiuretic hor-
 mone
Volatile acid, 125

W

Water
 filtration, excretion and reabsorption of, 50*t*
 reabsorption; *see* Sodium chloride and water reabsorp-
 tion
Water balance disorders, 70
Water channels, 76
Water permeability
 actions of ADH on, 75-76, 83